The H. L. Mencken Baby Book

The H. L. Mencken Baby Book

Comprising the Contents of H. L. Mencken's
What You Ought to Know About Your Baby
with commentaries

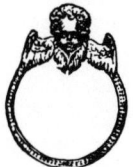

Howard Markel, M.D.   •   Frank A. Oski, M.D.

HANLEY & BELFUS, INC.
Philadelphia

Publisher: HANLEY & BELFUS, INC.
              210 S. 13th Street
              Philadelphia, PA 19107
              (215) 546-7293

Copyright © 1990 by Hanley & Belfus, Inc.

All rights reserved. No part of this book may be reproduced, reused, republished, or transmitted in any form or by any means without written permission of the publisher.

Library of Congress Cataloging-in-Publication Data
Mencken, H. L. (Henry Louis), 1880–1956.
 The H. L. Mencken baby book.
 1. Child care.   I. Markel, Howard.   II. Oski, Frank A.
                        III. Title.
                  RJ61.M558   1989
649′.122   89-20104

The H. L. Mencken Baby Book
ISBN 0-932883-22-2

Designed by Adrianne Onderdonk Dudden
Printed in the United States of America
9 8 7 6 5 4 3 2 1

To Deborah Gordin Markel (1958–1988)

"Age cannot wither her, nor custom stale
Her infinite variety…"

William Shakespeare, *Antony and Cleopatra* (II, ii, 243)

Contents

What You Ought to Know About
What You Ought to Know About Your Baby 1

1 The Slaughter of the Innocents 27
2 The New-Born Baby 45
3 Baby's First Few Months 56
4 The Nursing Baby 65
5 Mother and Baby 74
6 The Bottle-Fed Baby 85
7 A Chapter on Milk 89
8 The Food for Growing Children 105
9 What You Ought to Know About Your School 111
10 Need Every Child Have Catching Diseases? An Introduction to the Infectious and Communicable Diseases 125
11 If Your Baby Had Diphtheria 135
12 If Your Baby Had Scarlet Fever 145
13 Whooping Cough: It Kills More Than Diphtheria and Scarlet Fever Together 156
14 If Your Baby Had Pneumonia 165
15 Need Every Child Have Measles? 174

Notes 185
Index 187

Preface

If one were challenged to list the most unlikely authors of a baby book, H. L. Mencken should soon appear, perhaps just following W. C. Fields. Eventually Theodore Dreiser, who was said by his biographer, W. A. Swanberg, to have "loved children in the abstract so long as he did not have to deal with them in his own household," would be mentioned, at least by the literati. Yet, over the summer of 1907 these two men formed a most unlikely troika with a physician named Leonard K. Hirshberg—of the three the most unsavory role model for a child—to enlighten the American public on the care and feeding of infants. The mutual friendships and working relationship that developed from this publishing venture would influence not only child rearing but the course of American literature.

The fact that the book that eventually resulted, *What You Ought to Know About Your Baby,* was almost entirely written by Mencken is not well known, even by most Mencken scholars. The book was released with Leonard Keene Hirshberg, B.A., M.D. as sole author in order to enhance its credibility with mothers. However, anyone familiar with Mencken's style will immediately recognize the true identity of the author.

In this book we have reproduced *What You Ought to Know About Your Baby* in its entirety. In addition, we have introduced new material to establish both the literary and medical circumstances in which it was written, and we have prepared updated answers, based on the modern study of pediatrics, to the questions at the end of chapters where appropriate. The original questions and answers represent the only written contribution of Hirshberg. He based these on Mencken's text and often used the journalist's prose in the answers. Because medicine and science have revolutionized the management of infectious diseases, it did not seem to serve a purpose to update the answers to the final six chapters.

We hope that this book will interest not only readers of Mencken and Dreiser, but also contemporary pediatricians and parents, who should benefit from this unusual review of the progress of infant and child care in the 20th century.

Howard Markel, M.D.
Frank A. Oski, M.D.
Baltimore, Maryland

Authors and Acknowledgments

Howard Markel, the first-named author of this book, came to Baltimore to begin his internship in pediatrics at the Johns Hopkins Hospital in July 1986. Shortly thereafter his affection for Henry Louis Mencken led him to the Enoch Pratt Free Library and its lush H. L. Mencken collection. It was there that he discovered three rarely opened copies of *What You Ought to Know About Your Baby,* each autographed by Mencken. Additional research on the development of the book, including access to Mencken's papers and letters, was greatly assisted by Messrs. Neil Jordahl, Vincent Fitzpatrick, and Wilbur McGill at the Pratt. The text of *What You Ought to Know About Your Baby* is reprinted with the permission of the Enoch Pratt Free Library in accordance with the terms of the will of H. L. Mencken.

Dr. Frank A. Oski, the second-named author, is Chairman of Pediatrics at Johns Hopkins and oversaw the preparation of this work. He helped to update the question and answer sections of the original chapters.

Dr. Jean-Maurice Poitras, doubtless the world's leading expert on the life and career of Leonard Keene Hirshberg, was both generous and instructive in sharing his Hirshberg materials. Similarly, the authors are grateful to Laurel Blewett of the Johns Hopkins Hospital Pediatrics Library; the staff of the William H. Welch Medical Library, Johns Hopkins University; the staff of the Special Collections, Van Pelt Library, University of Pennsylvania, where The Theodore Dreiser Collection is stored; and the staff of the Butterick Company Archives, New York City.

The authors would also like to thank Lori Waugh, who patiently transcribed the handwritten manuscript into a typed one; the Harriet Lane pediatric house staff at the Johns Hopkins Hospital; the H.L.

Mencken Society; and Drs. Gert Breiger, Catherine DeAngelis, and Jane Oski of the Johns Hopkins Hospital, and Drs. Horace Davenport and Arthur Vander of the University of Michigan, who reviewed the manuscript. Above all, the first author would like to thank his late wife, Debby Markel, who provided him with unflagging love and support throughout the preparation of this work.

What You Ought to Know About *What You Ought to Know About Your Baby*

The Collaboration of H. L. Mencken, Dr. Leonard K. Hirshberg, and Theodore Dreiser

Over the summer of 1907, a magazine editor, a doctor, and a reporter joined forces to explain the care and feeding of infants. This topic was addressed in a series of magazine articles that were then expanded into a collected work entitled *What You Ought to Know About Your Baby*. The authors were two Baltimoreans: Dr. Leonard Keene Hirshberg, a 1902 graduate of the Johns Hopkins Medical School and a local practitioner, and Henry Louis Mencken, then an associate editor for the *Baltimore Sun* and on the brink of his tumultuous rise to becoming, as described by Walter Lippmann, "the most powerful personal influence on this whole generation of educated people."[1] The vehicle for this literary enterprise was *The Delineator*, one of three monthly magazines published by the Butterick Company, a firm that sold tissue-paper patterns of the latest dress fashions. Butterick's editor-in-chief was none other than Theodore Dreiser, about whom Mencken was later to say, "No other man had greater influence upon my youth."[2] Dreiser solicited the baby care articles from Mencken and Hirshberg during his editorial tenure at Butterick; he also cultivated and nurtured a friendship with H.L. Mencken that was to serve both writers' careers well throughout their lives. Although it seems difficult to believe that advice on baby care was the initial artistic project that brought Mencken and Dreiser together, the fact is that *What You Ought to Know About Your Baby* launched this provocative literary partnership.

The Delineator Magazine

The Butterick Company manufactures dress patterns—more dress patterns than any other single company in the world. Its beginnings, like those of most companies, were humble. In 1863 a Massachusetts tailor named Ebenezer Butterick, on the advice of his wife, applied for and received a United States patent on his tissue-type paper dress patterns. The Buttericks began manufacturing and selling the patterns locally shortly thereafter. Coinciding with the invention of the sewing machine by Elias Howe in 1846, Isaac Singer's subsequent development of the continuous-stitch sewing machine in 1851, and an era when most women practiced home dressmaking, E. Butterick and Company soon became wildly successful.

By 1902, when the firm was reorganized by its chief executive, George Wilder, Butterick was producing millions of dress patterns a year. Headquartered in its own 15-story "skyscraper" on Spring and MacDougal Streets in New York, the Butterick Company operated 86 printing presses and consumed tons of paper daily to accommodate its vast output of dress patterns, advertisements, and periodicals. The sheer volume of printed matter produced by Butterick was second only to the U.S. Government Printing Office in Washington D.C., the world's largest publishing organization.

Among the Butterick publications were three monthly magazines, *The Delineator, The Designer,* and *New Idea Women's Magazine.* These publications served the company as vehicles for advertising its dress patterns. *The Delineator* was the flagship of this trio and in 1904 had approximately 1 million readers. A typical issue at the turn of the century devoted the first 50 pages exclusively to detailed and breathtaking drawings of various dress fashions of the day, which could be ordered by the reader as a Butterick dress pattern for 10 to 15 cents each. The magazine, however, was old-fashioned in concept in contrast to many other periodicals of the Progressive Era (1901–1919). For example, magazines such as *McClure's, Collier's,* and the *American Magazine* were busy exposing corruption in the business and political worlds. Muckraking journalists such as Ida Tarbell, nemesis to the Rockefellers and the Standard Oil Company; Upton Sinclair, who exposed the filthy conditions of the Chicago stockyards and meatpacking plants in his serialized novel *The Jungle;* Samuel Hopkins Adams, who uncovered forms of medical quackery; and a host of others were at the height of their power. Simply put, all practices that affected the lives of private citizens were vulnerable to exposure by the muckrakers. *The Delineator*, on the other hand, like the Butterick dress patterns it advertised, was conservative and safe. In keeping with the magazine's motto "Safe Fashions for Home People," *The Delineator* would be recommended by a mother to her daughter without reservation. Arthur Sullivant Hoffman, who served as Butterick's managing editor under Dreiser, best described *The Delineator* as "fashion sheet with an omelet of magazine material around it... [intended] for rural and small-town women, as well as their displaced sisters in the city."[3]

The Editor: Theodore Dreiser

Theodore Dreiser, who was born in Terre Haute in 1871 and grew up in Indiana, began his literary career as a journeyman reporter in Chicago and then St. Louis. He drifted from job to job before trying his hand at fiction, following which he produced the manuscript of his first novel, *Sister Carrie*, in 1899. The novel chronicles the life of Carrie Meeber, who flees the stifling life of a small farming community for the excitement of the "big city," Chicago. Throughout the novel Dreiser reveals his understanding of and sensitivity for the woman who desired more from life than being a good cook and housekeeper. The writer also appreciates that a woman of that time had to focus on the domestic values of home and family in order to function free of any suspicion of scandal. Carrie forsakes the values of marriage, children, and maintaining a good home to live out of wedlock with one man and then another. Despite the protagonist's wicked ways, Carrie rises to great success as an actress, revealing Dreiser's rejection of the prevailing view of the sanctity of domesticity.

Frank Doubleday, president of the publishing house of Doubleday and Page, accepted Dreiser's manuscript for publication but was plagued with second thoughts about the then risqué novel. The firm decided to back out of publishing *Sister Carrie* gracefully and offered Dreiser the plates of the novel in return for releasing the company from its obligations. A major battle ensued between the obstreperous Dreiser and the publishing house, with the final result of Doubleday and Page publishing rather unenthusiastically one of the seminal American novels of the century. Receiving little advertising and backing from Doubleday, the book sold poorly, and Dreiser remained embittered against the firm until the day he died, embellishing with each telling his version of how Doubleday and Page abused America's greatest literary giant.

Shortly after the *Sister Carrie* debacle, Dreiser experienced what is labelled generically in the literature as a "nervous breakdown." Unable to write or concentrate, he became depressed and contemplated suicide. Although trying to compose *Jennie Gerhardt*, a novel Mencken would later review as "the best American novel I have ever read, with the lonesome but Himalayan exception of *Huckleberry Finn*,"[4] he was having little success. In need of money and work, Dreiser returned to the journalistic arena in 1904 as an assistant feature editor of Frank Munsey's *New York Daily News*. Soon after that, in 1905, he took a job as editor of *Smith's Magazine*, and then *Broadway Magazine* from 1906 to 1907, having great success at both by increasing circulation and improving style. His success with *Broadway Magazine* was particularly spectacular, with a reviewer calling the magazine under Dreiser's editorship "the prettiest piece of transformation work seen in New York for many a day."[5]

In early 1907 George Wilder, president of the Butterick Publications Company, was searching for a new editor-in-chief of the company's periodicals. The previous editor had committed suicide in a romantic fit over a failed love affair. Wilder wrote to Dreiser at his *Broadway* office (misspelling the writer's name as "Dreyser") on June 6, 1907, asking him to call the Butterick offices the following morning.[6] Dreiser, having grown dissatisfied with the management of *Broadway* and eager to work for a concern as profitable and large as Butterick, met with Wilder. Dreiser left Wilder's 15th floor office with a contract to edit the three Butterick magazines at an astronomical salary, by 1907 standards, of $7,000 a year, plus bonuses for increasing circulation.

Although under Dreiser's command *The Delineator* was to remain "a fashion sheet with an omelet of magazine around it," the omelet was soon to be enriched with a variety of features and articles that would appeal to the women readers as well as carry important but uncontroversial social messages of the day. One of Dreiser's first editorials in *The Delineator* stated, with the grandiloquence of a seasoned public relations artist, the goals and directions of the magazine under his editorship:

> A magazine's greatness is determined by one thing alone, its message. *The Delineator's* message is human betterment. Its appeal is to the one great humanizing force of humanity—womanhood. To sustain it, to broaden it, to refine it, is our aim. Our theme is one that a woman may carry into her home, her church and her social affairs—the theme of the ready smile, the theme of the ungrudged helping hand.[7]

In direct contrast to the views he expressed in *Sister Carrie*, Dreiser continued to wave the flag of wholesome, virtuous, American motherhood throughout his tenure at Butterick. He adopted the muckraker's techniques, however, in his advocacy of child welfare by publishing numerous articles in *The Delineator* about orphanages, health care issues, and related subjects. In many respects, Dreiser's public campaigns for child welfare and the ideals of home and family were highly representative of the way that issues regarding children were dealt with during the Progressive Era. Historian Nancy Pottishman Weiss referred to the Progressive view of childhood as a "bifurcated vision," consisting of public, group-oriented movements dedicated to reforming the schools and playgrounds, to the institution of public recreational facilities and juvenile courts, and to the establishment of protective child labor laws. The other vision was more private and was characterized by "preoccupation with children in the home and a growing stress on the application of science to child rearing."[8] Dreiser was to fulfill both visions with his child rescue campaigns, advocacy for children's rights and health, and, on a more private home-based scale, his promotion of a baby book that would teach mothers how to care for their children using the expert advice of physicians.

Dreiser began his child rescue work by running a poignant story by Mabel Porter Daggett entitled "The Child Without a Home," which appeared in the October 1907 issue of *The Delineator*. The article discussed the Dickensian plight of homeless children at the New York Foundling Hospital. Dreiser, who was said to have "loved children in the abstract so long as he did not have to deal with them in his own household,"[9] quickly saw the appeal these innocent orphans held for his readers. He proceeded to design a plan to fund local orphan homes and to encourage adoptions by running a monthly feature on two or three beautifully presented, wistful-eyed waifs who needed a home. After the first month's appearance of *The Delineator's* Child Rescue Campaign in November 1907, the response from the readers was so great that the editor found homes for many more orphans than he had room in his magazine to profile. Publisher George Wilder, too, thought that such a campaign would not only benefit the orphans but also his company's receipts and urged Dreiser to press forward.

The Delineator's Child Rescue Campaign, which immediately received the accolades of prominent women such as Mrs. Edith Rockefeller McCormick, Mrs. Frederick Dent Grant, and Mrs. William Jennings Bryan, was to continue for three years under Dreiser's devoted and active command. Along the way Theodore Dreiser received extensive newspaper coverage for his work and saw *The Delineator's* circulation rise to the 2 million mark. Dreiser's national crusade for child welfare became so celebrated that he was invited to meet with President Theodore Roosevelt in 1908, presenting the Rough Rider with a "mass of data which disclosed that thousands upon thousands of children throughout the country are found to be in a deplorable state simply because they have been denied the home influences which are so necessary in a child's life."[10]

In fact, Dreiser, with the aid of Judge James H. West, met with President Roosevelt several times that year, resulting in the establishment of the first White House Conference on Children in January 1909. These meetings presaged and inspired the formation of the American Association for the Study and Prevention of Infant Mortality, the White House Conferences on Children (held each decade), and the nationally sponsored Children's Bureau, which in 1912 was charged by Congress "to investigate and report upon all matters pertaining to the welfare of children...."[11] Other programs and activities benefiting child welfare, such as the founding in 1909 of seven Butterick-sponsored schools for mothers in the tenement districts of New York, with nurses and physicians teaching feeding, food preparation, hygiene, and bottle care, and the incorporation of the New York Child Welfare Committee, were instigated by Dreiser through *The Delineator* magazine.[12]

With all of these projects in motion, it is not surprising that Dreiser and his publisher George Wilder decided to solicit and publish in *The Delineator* a series of articles on baby care and feeding by Mencken and Hirshberg. From the beginning Wilder had great plans for such a series, planning to re-issue the articles in book form under the patronage of the Butterick Company. In response to Dreiser's "If I Were Santa Claus" feature, a series that appeared in *The Delineator's* 1908 Christmas issue and revealed what notable people might like to do for children if they were St. Nicholas, Wilder himself wished:

> That the Health department in every city in this country be authorized to buy some one book on the care of children ... and give one copy to every mother on the birth of a child ... such books might cost the state 20 or 25 cents each. The lives thus saved — the children grown to healthy men and women, that under present conditions die in early youth or come up pallid, colorless, bloodless creatures, the germ of vitality killed at the beginning — would bring the State a return for such investments that it could never estimate.[13]

Wilder continued to be a strong influence on the proceedings of the "baby book" and carefully read each manuscript of the proposed articles by Mencken and Hirshberg. He often passed on to the writers, through Dreiser, memoranda about his own experiences with infant feeding, crying patterns, and other childhood behaviors. Much of this information, based upon Wilder's uncontrolled studies of the Wilder children, influenced advice promulgated in the pages of *What You Ought to Know About Your Baby*. Indeed, Wilder's influence on the book was so great that the authors dedicated it to him.

The Collaborators: H. L. Mencken and Leonard K. Hirshberg

As F. O. Matthiessen once mused, it is difficult to decide which writer was farther from his proper work: Mencken, a long-time, vociferous bachelor, actually writing about babies; or Dreiser, a ladies man so notorious he once excused himself between courses of dinner with his wife for a tete à tete with one of his lovers, actually soliciting the articles.[14] Mencken proudly proclaimed in his satiric treatise *In Defense of Women*:

> The marriage of a first rate man, when it takes place at all, commonly takes place relatively late. He may succumb in the end, but he is almost always able to postpone the disaster a good deal longer than the average poor clodpate, or normal man.[15]

True to his word, the Sage of Baltimore did not marry until 1930, at the age of 50, when he wed the southern writer Sara Powell Haardt, a woman 22 years his junior. The couple lived in a brownstone rowhouse overlooking Baltimore's Mt. Vernon Park and, ironically, next door to a Christian Science Church, a religion Mencken particularly enjoyed lampooning. The marriage, which produced no children, was marred by Sara's long struggle with tuberculosis which resulted in removal of a kidney in 1933 and her death from tuberculous meningitis in 1935.

Despite Mencken's carefully fostered reputation as a bachelor and a curmudgeon, he enjoyed children and often played with the poor black children living in the tenements behind his house. However, his only real experience with child-rearing and pediatrics was that he was once an infant himself—hardly the credentials necessary to author a baby book. Furthermore, Mencken had no formal training in medicine, despite his lifelong interest in the human body and pathology.

As a schoolboy, Mencken proved himself to be an able scholar. He was consistently praised during his grammar school years at the F. Knapp Institute as its best student. He received equal acclaim during high school at Baltimore Polytechnic. For example, young Mencken achieved a perfect score on his high school physiology final and maintained an active knowledge of the subject throughout his life. Chemistry and English were Mencken's favorite school subjects, and as a teenager he wavered between becoming a chemist and a writer. Fortunately for American literature, the choice was the pen instead of the test tube, although he continued to read and keep abreast of scientific and technical literature throughout adulthood. Mencken frequently showed off this knowledge by publicly commenting on advances of science, spicing his prose with scientific terms and concepts, and promoting the efforts of other writers to popularize science.

Mencken's formal education ended with high school. His father, August, offered him the opportunity to attend college at Johns Hopkins or, alternatively, matriculation at the University of Maryland Law School. The obstinate 18-year-old refused, declaring that he wanted newspaper work or nothing. Mencken evidently lost this battle with his father, for he went directly from the stage where he delivered his valedictory address at Baltimore Polytechnic to his father's cigar factory.[16] There, he rolled cigars and repressed his journalistic yearnings for 18 months. In January 1899, however, August Mencken developed a raging kidney infection that progressed to sepsis and death in a matter of weeks. Henry, who was ill himself with "a sore throat that stuck to me more or less steadily for 10 years," bronchitis, and what may have been tuberculosis, was shocked by his father's death but summoned enough courage to leave the cigar factory the day after the patriarch's burial. He applied for and received a staff position on the *Baltimore Morning Herald* after displaying a great deal of persistence and youthful enthusiasm. In essence, the city of Baltimore was to serve as Mencken's college, as he notes in the second volume of his memoirs, *Newspaper Days*:

> At a time when the respectable bourgeois youngsters of my generation were college freshman, oppressed by simian sophomores and affronted with balderdash daily and hourly by chalky pedagogues, I was at large in a wicked seaport with a front row seat at every public show, as free of the night as of the day, and getting earfuls and eyefuls of instruction in a hundred giddy arcana, none of them taught in schools.[17]

Mencken was extremely successful at the *Morning Herald*, rising from police reporter to city reporter to editor of the daily paper in 1905, when he was only 25. Work on a busy, metropolitan newspaper, the continuous exercise of finding interesting stories, and the meeting of thousands of deadlines proved to be quite an education in themselves.

Always the prolific wordsmith, Mencken began to supplement his income by writing articles for various magazines. In those days before the omnipresence of movies, radio, and television, the written word was, of course, a major source of entertainment. Then, as now, not all Americans had the ambition to struggle with a lengthy novel or book of substance after a long day's work. Such a situation created a huge market for what were known as pulp novels and magazines. Called pulp because they were printed on the cheapest paper available, the novels were as sensational as the day allowed; the magazines were collections of lurid journalistic pieces and racy stories based on fact but often altered to sell more copies. It was a common occurrence for a dime-novel or two or three pulp magazines to serve as an evening's entertainment.

In his early twenties, Mencken began writing short stories and poems for periodicals such as *Leslie's Illustrated Monthly, Everybody's, Bookman*, the *New England Magazine*, and other now-forgotten magazines. He soon grew tired of fiction and began to appreciate, following the encouragement of his editors, that his literary flair lay in the form of the essay and factual articles. In a fascinating unpublished manuscript entitled "Autobiographical Notes," which Mencken compiled in 1925 for Isaac Goldberg's biography *The Man Mencken*, he briefly describes how he came to dabble in medical journalism:

> There was in those days a demand among magazines for medical articles and one day Sedgwick [Ellery Sedgwick, editor of *Leslie's Magazine*]

asked me to find a man at Johns Hopkins who would be willing to write them for *Leslie's Monthly*. I discovered such a man in Dr. Leonard K. Hirshberg. Hirshberg was a fellow of great intelligence with an excellent medical education. He put down the facts and I wrote the articles. The combination turned out to be very successful and pretty soon we were deluged with orders. Among the magazines we worked for was *The Delineator*, then edited by Dreiser. Dreiser ordered a whole series of articles on the feeding and care of children. Hirshberg supplied the material and I did the writing. The series was afterward published as a book under the title of "What You Ought to Know About the Baby," or something of the sort, and under Hirshberg's name. The fact that I wrote it has never, as far as I know, got out.[18]

Most likely, Mencken met Hirshberg in the context of a patient consulting a physician. Leonard Hirshberg was born in Baltimore on 581 North Gay Street, a predominantly working-class, Jewish neighborhood, in 1877. He studied a typical premedical curriculum at the Johns Hopkins University and applied to the Johns Hopkins Medical School on September 20, 1898. William Henry Welch, then dean of the medical school and responsible for everything from research to reading applications, approved Hirshberg's admission.[19]

Having attended Johns Hopkins Medical School during its golden days, Hirshberg enjoyed what many considered to be the hallmark of American medical education. Between 1898 and 1902, Hirshberg learned anatomy from Franklin Mall, pharmacology from John J. Abel, and attended the clinics of internist William Osler, surgeon William Halsted, and gynecologist Howard Kelly. The list of the faculty at that time reads like a medical hall of fame. But although Hirshberg was a competent student, it is safe to state he was not at the top of his class. In those days, the medical students graduating from Hopkins with the best grade-point averages were offered a coveted Johns Hopkins Hospital internship. The best student could choose among medicine, surgery, pathology, gynecology, and obstetrics. There were about 13 positions in these fields open each year. The second-best student had the choice of the resident positions remaining, and so on down the line until all the positions were filled. It was not uncommon for a student to accept a different field of specialization simply to remain at Johns Hopkins. Hirshberg was passed over for this distinction and instead went abroad, which was a popular practice in that day, to further his education. He attended the well-known clinics in Berlin and Heidelberg. It is difficult to ascertain what Hirshberg learned in Europe, but the training probably was not as rigorous as the traditional Johns Hopkins Hospital internship. It seems likely the young doctor spent his days attending lectures at his leisure and his nights drinking German beer—an enjoyable sojourn but hardly the background necessary to declare oneself an expert on the diseases of children.

Upon returning to Baltimore in 1903, he became associated with the now-defunct Baltimore College of Physicians and Surgeons as an instructor in Bacteriology and Nervous Diseases and opened a practice in the fashionable neighborhood of Bolton Hill. Hirshberg's scholarly looks, a Teutonic beard and sideburns, pince-nez glasses, and a friendly demeanor soon made him a popular and busy general practitioner. By 1904 he was seeing between 50 and 60 adult patients a day in addition to writing a large number of scientific papers, mostly case reports or findings of no great import, for journals ranging from the *Maryland State Medical Journal* and the *Journal of the American Medical Association* to more obscure periodicals no longer in existence. Fulton Oursler, then a Baltimore newspaperman, who subsequently went on to great fame with his best seller *The Greatest Story Ever Told*, recalled Hirshberg in his 1964 autobiography *Behold This Dreamer!*:

> There lived in Baltimore in those days a fantastic figure, Dr. Leonard Keene Hirshberg, a five-foot man with voluptuous brown mustache and chinwhiskers, and bald head slashed with a great jagged scar (which he declared he had received in a duel with a student at Heidelberg). He was a graduate of Johns Hopkins University and the medical school and professor of clinical diseases at the hospital [the latter is absolutely false, as Hirshberg never held an appointment at either the Hospital or Medical School]. He was, at once, the friendliest man I have ever met—and perhaps the most amoral. He could have been a figure in medicine in those great Hopkins days, when Gildersleeve and Kelly and Welch and Osler were still living forces and the name of Hopkins stood for all that was eminent in the art of healing. But Hirshberg had skill and far too much facility and two great worldly itches: one to escape his wife and boys and dance with the youngest girls; and second, to be an author.[20]

One of the many papers Hirshberg published in 1904 was an article entitled "Antitoxin for Hay Fever and Rose Cold,"[21] describing an interesting serum treatment for hay fever, which Hirshberg later admitted did not work. Coincidentally, Mencken was a long-time sufferer of hay fever and chronic sinusitis, probably his most significant health problem until a tragic stroke in 1948 left him with global aphasia. He was obsessed with finding a cure or means of relief, in those pre-antihistamine days, for the condition that made him weepy-eyed and caused his nose to drip from spring to fall throughout his life. Indeed, Mencken kept a detailed journal year after year, preserved in the Mencken Collection at the Enoch Pratt Free Library in Baltimore, of the hay fever symptoms he experienced each summer. In these journals, he fanatically recorded his daily temperatures, aches and pains, and how many handkerchiefs he went through that day. He kept detailed notes on all of his medical complaints, and his papers collected at the Pratt Library include hundreds of cancelled checks made out to various physicians and surgeons.

As noted previously, Mencken was an avid follower of medical progress over a long period of time. He not only read medical textbooks and journals but also was friendly with many physicians in Baltimore including those who staffed the Johns Hopkins Hospital. His capitulation to hypochondriasis, as evidenced by his compulsive diaries of hay fever symptoms, extended to comparing remedies and even methods of anesthesia with friends such as the Johns Hopkins biostatistician Raymond Pearl, and listing his medical problems to George Jean Nathan, which included "a burn on the tongue (healing), a pimple inside the jaw, a sour stomach, a pain in the prostate, a burning in the gospel pipe, a cut finger, a small pimple inside the nose (going away), a razor cut (smarting), and tired eyes."[22] It seems likely, therefore, that he read or heard about Hirshberg's proposed hay fever cure and consulted the physician in late 1904 or early 1905. In fact, Mencken continued to see Hirshberg, professionally, on and off for the next 5 years, even submitting to a uvulectomy performed by the doctor in 1909. Mencken and Hirshberg apparently became friendly, sharing interests in music, German beer, and medicine, and while their initial meeting did not result in a cure for Mencken's hay fever, it did bring about their collaborative writing efforts.

For Hirshberg, collaboration with a newspaperman and the chance to achieve fame and fortune from writing made the venture ideal. For Mencken, the partnership was an opportunity to make money. The team began by writing an article entitled "Popular Medical Fallacies," which appeared in the *American Magazine's* October 1906 issue. The essay attempts to expose the myths associated with various maladies, including boils, colds, and nosebleeds, in a style that is undoubtedly Mencken's. For example, here is the description of phagocytosis (the process by which a cell envelops a foreign particle) and inflammation:

> Scientifically, all of this redness and heat and pain may be described as a battle between the intruding germs and the white corpuscles of your blood. As soon as the germs get into the skin the corpuscles attack them and try to swallow them. If you were to cut open a boil you would see the process plainly... Every now and then you will notice a white corpuscle approaches and gathers in a germ, just as an oyster swallows a baby crab.[23]

A second article for the *American Magazine*, entitled "Cancer, the Unconquered Plague," appeared in February 1907.[24] The review was a popular compendium on the various theories of the causes and possible cures for cancer proposed in the early 20th century. Both articles had only Hirshberg's name on the by-line and this was to be practiced throughout their collaboration.

As with any successful business venture, Mencken and Hirshberg were offering a product that was in great demand. The Progressive Era and its reforms kept the American public conscious of the need for progress. Indeed, science was equated with this sense of progress. Consequently, great public interest in the preventive medicine movement was generated; the movement advocated the use of science and medicine to prolong life and avoid disease, helped formulate health legislation, such as the Food and Drug Act of 1906, and inspired active scientific investigation. The lay public, too, wanted to keep abreast of medical and scientific issues that affected their lives. The monthly magazines, a major source of information and entertainment for Americans, scrambled to provide their readers with such articles. Soon, Mencken and Hirshberg were deluged with offers to write about health care topics.

The Book: *What You Ought to Know About Your Baby*

One of these offers was from Theodore Dreiser who, after reading the *American Magazine* pieces, asked Leonard Hirshberg to compose an article on child care for mothers. At the time, Dreiser did not know that Mencken was Hirshberg's collaborator. In his capacity as editorial director of a small publishing company, B.W. Dodge and Co., Dreiser had contacted Mencken at about the same time about the possibility of Mencken's preparing an edition of some German philosopher or dramatist for sale to schools and the general reading public, but he did not connect Mencken with Hirshberg.[25] Dreiser had probably become aware of Mencken through the journalist's published critical analyses of George Bernard Shaw and Friedrich Nietzche. In fact, Dreiser did not know of Mencken's relationship with Hirshberg until the fall of 1907, when he received the manuscript of an article entitled "'The Slaughter of the Innocents' by Leonard Keene Hirshberg" from Mencken. The essay discussed medical fallacies related to child care and warnings to mothers on the importance of assistance from a qualified pediatrician. Dreiser enjoyed the piece a great deal and quickly wrote to Mencken on September 24, 1907, asking him if he worked on the medical articles with Dr. Hirshberg and requesting two similar essays about pneumonia and diphtheria. Dreiser also complimented Hirshberg's writing style and his ability to convey medical advice in written form to mothers.[26] This compliment was Mencken's alone to receive, since the prose of the article was his own.

The team received $100 for their first essay, "The Slaughter of the Innocents," $125 for the article on pneumonia, and $125 for the diphtheria essay. The two writers split the fees they earned fifty-fifty, just as they shared the work: Hirshberg would look up the subject at hand, usually relying on major textbooks, and provide the facts for

Mencken, who subsequently put them into readable and entertaining prose. The by-line was Hirshberg's, however, because the writing team agreed that "Leonard K. Hirshberg, A.B., A.M., M.D. (The Johns Hopkins University)," as he was to sign all his articles, would substantiate medical advice more than Mencken's.

Fortunately, Theodore Dreiser recorded his memories of his first meeting with H.L. Mencken some 18 years after the event. Dreiser, however, confuses his dates a bit, and it is important to preface Dreiser's version with Mencken's acerbic comment "the one thing Dreiser hated was a fact":

> It was sometime during the Spring or Summer of 1908, and my second year of editorial control of the Butterick Publications, that there came to me a doctor by the name of Leonard K. Hirshberg, who explained that besides being a physician of some practice in Baltimore he was a graduate of Johns Hopkins and interested in interpreting to the lay public if possible the more recent advances in medical knowledge. There had been various recent developments, as there always are. Some phases of these he proposed to describe in articles of various lengths. And then it was that he announced that, being a medical man and better equipped technically in that line than as a writer, he had joined with a newspaper man or editorial writer then connected with the *Baltimore Sun*, Henry L. Mencken. The name being entirely unfamiliar to me at the time, he proceeded to describe him as a young, refreshing and delightful fellow of a very vigorous and untechnical skill, who, in combination with himself, would most certainly be able to furnish me with articles of exceptional luminosity and vigor. Liking two or three of the subjects discussed, I suggested that between them they prepare one and submit it. In case it proved satisfactory, I would buy it and possibly some of the others.
>
> In less than three weeks thereafter I received a discussion of some current medical development which seemed to me as refreshing and colorful a bit of semi-scientific exposition as I had read in years. While setting forth all the developments which had been indicated to me, it bristled with gay phraseology and a largely suppressed though still peeping mirth. I was so pleased that I immediately wrote Hirshberg that the material was satisfactory and that I would be willing to contract with him and his friend for one of the other subjects he mentioned.[27]

The article explaining pneumonia, an extremely serious cause of infant mortality and morbidity in 1908, was so well-received by *Delineator* readers that Dreiser became quite eager to publish more of the same. Curiously, however, the diphtheria essay never appeared in *The Delineator*. Although Mencken and Dreiser had frequently corresponded, Dreiser was anxious to meet the young reporter who was ghost-writing Hirshberg's articles and invited him to visit the Butterick offices on March 9, 1908.[28]

And then some weeks later in connection with that or some other matter, whether to discuss it more fully or merely to deliver it or to make the acquaintance of the man who was interested in this new literary combination, there appeared in my office a taut, ruddy, blue-eyed, snub-nosed youth of twenty eight or nine whose brisk gait and ingratiating smile proved to me at once enormously intriguing and amusing. I had, for some reason not connected to his basic mentality you may be sure, the sense of a small town roisterer or a college sophomore of the crudest and yet most disturbing charm and imp-ishness, who, for some reason, had strayed into the field of letters. More than anything he reminded me of a spoiled and petted and possibly overfinanced brewer's or wholesale grocer's son who was out for a lark. With the sang-froid of a Caesar or a Napoleon he made himself comfortable in a large and impressive chair which was designed primarily to reduce the over-confidence of the average beginner. And from that particular and unintended vantage point he beamed on me with the confidence of a smirking fox about to devour a chicken. So I was the editor of the Butterick Publications. He had been told about me. However, in spite of *Sister Carrie*, I doubt if he had ever heard of me before this. After studying him in that almost arch-episcopal setting which the chair provided, I began to laugh. "Well, well," I said, "If it isn't Anheuser's own brightest boy out to see the town." And with that unfailing readiness for any nonsensical flight that has always charac-terized him, he proceeded to insist that this was true. "Certainly he was Baltimore's richest brewer's son and the yellow shoes and bright tie he was wearing were characteristic of the jack-dandies and rowdy-dows of his native town. Why not. What else did I expect? His father brewed the best beer in the world." All thought of the original purpose of the conference was at once dismissed and instead we proceeded to palaver and yoo-hoo anent the more general phrases and ridiculosities of life, with the result that an understanding based on a mutual liking was established, and from then on I counted him among those whom I most prized—temperamentally as well as intellectually. And to this day, despite various disagreements, that mood has never varied.[29]

In June 1908, Dreiser had contracted Hirshberg and Mencken, at the urging of Butterick president George Wilder, to a "series of six articles containing practical advice to the mother on the care and feeding of infants from birth until 3 or 5 years of age, or whenever it is that the infant stage ends."[30] Dreiser was wiling to pay $60.00 per article and wanted them to be only 1800 to 2000 words in length. The editor also stipulated that he wanted the rights to reproduce the articles in pamphlet or book form for distribution to mothers in keeping with George Wilder's 1908 Santa Claus wish. Mencken responded positively and promised to send word to Hirshberg about the project. The usually overconfident Mencken, however, voiced some concerns about writing such a book that would be understand-able and informative.[31]

Mencken and Hirshberg, with the input of Wilder, had determined an outline for the series, which Dreiser titled "What You Ought to Know About Your Baby," in early December 1908. It was to begin with articles on "The Newborn Baby and Its First Few Months," "The Nursing Baby," and "The Food of the Growing Baby and the Bottle Fed Baby." Further topics to be discussed included:

1. The baby at birth, its height, habits, and how to care for it. Common fallacies. How to detect abnormalities.
2. The care of a very young infant. Teething. Sleeping, crying [a subject that held great interest for George Wilder], feeding, drinking, and cautions regarding medicines and dressing.
3. The formation of habits in the child. The dawning of intelligence. Exercise and airing.
4. Natural methods of feeding the infant. Artificial foods.
5. The year-old baby and its care.
6. The second summer and afterward.[32]

A total of ten baby care articles by Mencken and Hirshberg appeared on an almost monthly basis in *The Delineator* between August 1908 and October 1909. These magazine articles and an additional five essays on nutrition and contagious diseases appeared in book form in 1910 under the title *What You Ought to Know About Your Baby: A Textbook for Mothers on the Care and Feeding of Babies, with Questions and Answers Especially Prepared by the Editor*. The book was published and distributed by the Butterick Company. It is difficult to ascertain just how many copies were produced, since it was distributed free of charge to anyone writing to Butterick for a copy. However, the book enjoyed reasonable popularity, went through several printings, and continued to be issued by Butterick until 1923, when the copyright was turned over to Leonard Hirshberg.

The factual information in the text was based almost entirely upon the experience and writings of a qualified pediatrician, Luther Emmett Holt. Holt was Professor of Pediatrics at New York's College of Physicians and Surgeons and Attending Physician at Babies Hospital. As director of the financially unstable Babies Hospital, in 1889 Holt found himself in the middle of a severe nursing shortage and without the funds to hire more help. At the suggestion of Mrs. Robert Chapin, he hired, with a minimum of expense, young girls who would serve in the capacity of "nursery maids." These women extended the services of the few trained graduate nurses at Babies Hospital and learned proper infant care from them. Once the nursery maids had completed the specified training and education, they were issued a diploma endorsed by Dr. Holt, attesting to their skills.

The course Holt prescribed was at first 4 to 6 months in length and included hands-on care of the hospital's young patients in addition to formal lectures in infant feeding and nursery hygiene. The nursery maid school program was a great success and the number of applicants continued to grow each year. In order to streamline the teaching process, Holt composed a booklet he called *A Catechism for Nurses,* "in which questions were asked and answered about bathing, feeding, sleep, fresh air, and so on."[33] The nursing students were required to study and memorize the catechism and upon graduation took their copies with them to spread Dr. Holt's gospel at their new nursery posts. Soon several others involved in infant care wrote to Holt requesting copies of his booklet in order to emulate the nursery maid school program at Babies Hospital. The demand for copies of the booklet became so great that Holt published it in 1894 as a book entitled *The Care and Feeding of Children.* The book eventually grew to a length of 200 pages and went through 12 revisions during the author's life, including 75 printings, and translations in Spanish, Russian, and Chinese. It remained an extremely popular source of information on infant care well into the 1940s and continued to be edited and revised by L. Emmett Holt, Jr. after his father's death. Indeed, the Grolier Club of America selected the book in 1946 for its list of 100 titles that "influenced the life and culture of American people." Further, the New York *World* noted, in a review of this book, "if women were not permitted to marry until they could pass a fair examination in this short catechism...the death rate would be decreased at least one-third."[35]

Just what did Dr. L. Emmett Holt prescribe that made him so popular among American mothers from the 1890s well into the 1940s? Holt, like most pediatricians of his day, advocated strict, regimented care of the infant "with no more coddling."[36] In Holt's view, the mother was the dominant figure in the mother/child relationship and she should assert that dominance freely. The infant's every action was to be directed by the parents, and this stern approach included toilet training by age 3 to 4 months. Children's hospitals during this time emphasized the importance of control over a child's behavior and daily activities. For example, when an infant became ill and hospitalization was required, parents were not allowed to visit the baby, particularly if the disease was contagious. The child's hands were usually tied in restraints and little interaction with other children or nurturing adults was allowed. Holt also stressed the importance of parents relying upon the ultimate source of child care information, the pediatrician.

Holt's book appeared at a time when the public began to rely upon scientific principles and progress to improve the quality and length of life and address the glaring problem of infant mortality. Few experts could argue against Dr. Holt's uncompromising adherence to the importance of hygiene and the prevention of infection in an era when infant mortality was so high. Even Dr. Benjamin Spock, whose treatise on a more permissive style of child-rearing first appeared in 1945, was raised by his mother according to the strict precepts of Dr. Holt.[37]

George Wilder was well acquainted with Holt's book because he used it for advice in rearing his own children. Wilder often recommended Holt's book to new mothers and urged Mencken and Hirshberg to use the text as a reference for the Butterick-sponsored baby book, perhaps hoping for similar success. Many of the ideas and facts in *What You Ought to Know About Your Baby*, such as the avoidance of coddling an infant in order to prevent disease, the importance of relying upon an expert pediatrician's advice over that of one's neighbor or mother-in-law, and actual descriptions of infectious diseases, appeared first in Holt's baby book or were borrowed from Holt's textbook of pediatrics, *Diseases of Infancy and Childhood*. The addition of sections of questions and answers to the book version of *What You Ought to Know About Your Baby*, which represent the only passages of the book written solely by Hirshberg, was obviously based on Holt's successful "catechism" style.

While *What You Ought to Know About Your Baby* enjoyed popularity during the second decade of the 20th century, it hardly came close to the success of the book it so obviously imitated. The essays that comprise the text make for entertaining, accurate, and lively discourses on selected topics in child care, but it is not a book that one could rush to in the middle of the night for a quick answer about one's baby. Holt's baby book, and later Benjamin Spock's *Baby and Child Care*, were scrupulously indexed, comprehensive textbooks of child-rearing, making them as often found in the nursery as diapers or baby oil. For the new mother, the Mencken and Hirshberg book was a serviceable introduction to infant care and important health issues, but simply lacked the scope or length to become the "Bible" of baby care Holt's book was or Spock's book was to become. The book's strongest suit, however, is that no other book in the fields of infant care or medicine displays the acerbic and lively style of a writer as gifted as H.L. Mencken. Mencken's handling of such topics as breastfeeding, bottlefeeding, developmental pediatrics, and contagious diseases was not only accurate but humorous and literate. Furthermore, many of the positions Mencken was to take in later essays on medical matters, education and schooling, the perils of infancy, and the germ theory, to be discussed in the chapters to follow, first appeared in seminal form in *What You Ought to Know About Your Baby*.

After Mencken and Hirshberg ended their collaborative writing efforts with the publication of the baby book, Hirshberg continued to accept offers to write popular accounts of medical matters for a variety of sources. The physician became so prolific in his new-found trade that between 1907 and 1920 he wrote and published 30 papers for the medical literature, 50 articles for trade magazines (ranging from *Scientific American* and *Harper's* to *Ladies Home Journal*), a daily medical advice column for the Hearst chain of over 400 newspapers, and four books. Fulton Oursler recalls Hirshberg's transformation from physician to "literary factory" in his autobiography:

In an evil hour for him, Hirshberg wrote an article and sent it to the *American Magazine* and John S. Phillips bought the piece for four hundred dollars. To a young doctor, the fact that medical knowledge could earn him such a sum for a few hours' work was staggering...

Soon Hirshberg was no longer a doctor; he became a literary factory. His scheme was very simple: he engaged four stenographers—two blondes, a brunette, and a redhead, any one of them fit for the front line of a chorus—and every afternoon he would arrive with his entourage at the reading room of the Central Public Library. There the five of them would sit down at a round table; from the clerk, Leonard would then gather an armful of obscure and inconsequential scientific publications—reports of county medical societies, consular reports from the port cities of the world, things that nobody else bothered to read. These he would skim through until his eye fell upon a possibility. It might be, for example, a report from some unknown doctor in an unheard of county in Arizona, declaring that he had treated housemaid's knee with injections of snake venom and was sure he had discovered a cure. That was all that Hirshberg would need.[38]

Denouement

Leonard Hirshberg's prodigious literary output rapidly replaced medical practice as his major source of income. Yet his self-promotional tactics and blatant aspirations to fame and fortune soon grated on Mencken's less-than-tolerant nerves. This behavior also alienated him from Dreiser. In fact, almost every reference to Hirshberg in the Mencken-Dreiser correspondence from February 6, 1910 on is derogatory. The barbs range from pedestrian comments about Hirshberg's baldness to disturbing glimpses of Mencken's darker side, when he calls the doctor a "bumptious Jew" without tact.[39] Dreiser became particularly irritated at Hirshberg when he publicly offended the Italian medium Eusapia Palladino as she made her American debut in 1909. Dreiser, a long-time student and follower of the occult and supernatural, was anxious to meet with the highly touted medium and wanted to publicize her great powers in *The Delineator*.[40] Unfortunately, he invited Hirshberg to a party he was hosting in honor of Palladino and Hereward Carrington, a writer who had published an extensive study of Madame Eusapia. Hirshberg indelicately called the medium and her scribe frauds and demanded scientific proof of her alleged supernatural powers. To make matters worse, he sent the sensitive and perturbed Dreiser a letter in January 1910 offering $2000 to anyone who could perform Palladino's séance "tricks" under test conditions and the watchful eye of his self-appointed judges.[41] Hirshberg was relentless in his challenges against the medium and continued to annoy Dreiser with numerous letters and even a published article questioning the validity of Eusapia Palladino's powers.[42] Although other authorities, such as psychologist Hugo Munsterberg, had similarly accused Palladino of being a fraud, Dreiser was especially intolerant of such an attack from his friend Hirshberg. Dreiser became angrier and angrier with Hirshberg as the doctor's anti-Eusapia Palladino crusade escalated, to the point where he refused to answer Hirshberg's letters. For example, Dreiser wrote Mencken of his disgust with the physician in February 1910: "And as for Hirshberg, well the more I think of him the more I am sure he is punished enough. He has to live with himself."[43] Dreiser also refused to see Hirshberg and avoided visiting Baltimore in order to avoid a confrontation. When inviting Dreiser to Baltimore for crabs, Mencken made a point of promising Dreiser that Hirshberg would not pester him: "His effrontery growing painful, I have recently given him a rough settler."[44]

Mencken probably severed his relations with Hirshberg sometime in 1910. The last reference to Hirshberg in the Mencken-Dreiser correspondence is a letter from Mencken dated October 10, 1916. Mencken discussed a petition he was organizing to protest the suppression of Dreiser's novel *The Genius* by the Society for the Prevention of Vice and promised to omit a "few such lice as Hirshberg" from the list of signatures.[45]

Although Hirshberg lost favor with both Mencken and Dreiser, the critic and the novelist continued a symbiotic relationship that was to advance each other's career. Alas, Leonard Keene Hirshberg, was not to meet the illustrious fates of either his collaborator, Mencken, or his editor, Dreiser. His constant striving for attention and money, often at the expense of the truth, led him to become one of the most infamous physicians ever to graduate from Johns Hopkins.

Hirshberg's propensity to sensationalize medical half-truths and unsubstantiated quack cures first surfaced in 1912 when he published an article in *Popular Mechanics*,[46] claiming that the dermatologist W. Williams Lord had discovered a cure for leprosy. A second article published in the now-defunct *Technical World*[47] used illustrations from the internist W.S. Thayer's treatise on malaria, falsely identifying the malaria parasite as "cancer germs," and an unauthorized photograph of surgeon Joseph Bloodgood, identifying him as a German researcher. These three physicians, all faculty members of the Johns Hopkins Hospital and Medical School, were incensed at Hirshberg's blatant deceptions at their expense and in 1913 brought charges of impropriety against him to the Baltimore Medical Society and the Maryland Medical and Chiurgical Society. Hirshberg narrowly escaped the embarrassment of censure by resigning from these organizations after a messy court case based largely upon legal loopholes and chicanery.

Always signing his by-line "Leonard Keene Hirshberg, A.B., A.M., M.D. (Johns Hopkins University)," Hirshberg subtly misguided his readers into believing that the material that appeared below the by-line emanated from research at the medical institution. Hirshberg soon discovered that no medical topic was too mundane or outlandish to be turned into a publication. His articles ranged from discussions of bottlefeeding,[48] cancer,[49] and eye strain[50] to musings on how stoutness contributed to a tenor's voice;[51] one of his most ridiculous essays was a discourse on "Don, the Talking Dog."[52] Hirshberg's literary production line was to suspend operations in 1920, when he sought more lucrative prospects: investments in stocks, bonds, and real estate.

In the fall of 1921, Hirshberg became a managing partner in the stock brokerage house of Winthrop Smith and Company. The firm operated a "blind pool," a fund in which the customer places his money to be speculated at the discretion of the broker, with the broker receiving a percentage of the profits. In a series of pamphlets sent through the United States mail, Winthrop Smith and Company offered its investors a 120% return on their money. Not surprisingly, a large number of people took the company up on this incredible offer and soon business boomed at the firm's offices in New York, Baltimore, Cleveland, Schenectady, Elmira, and Harrisburg. By the following year, however, none of the company's 3000 investors had received a single dividend check, and the clients began to wonder exactly what the firm was doing with their money. A. U.S. Postal Service inquiry was instituted and found that Winthrop Smith, Leonard Hirshberg, and three other partners had bilked their investors out of 1 million dollars. Hirshberg and his associates were arrested for mail fraud on September 9, 1922, making the headlines almost daily until their conviction on May 2, 1923. True to form, Hirshberg and his attorneys attempted every last legal maneuver to avoid a jail sentence but, nevertheless, he was sentenced by Judge Learned Hand to four years in the Federal Penitentiary at Atlanta. Judge Hand called Hirshberg "the mastermind of the swindle."[53]

With his dynamic and outgoing personality, Hirshberg apparently made several lifelong friends, even if he was not nearly as successful in his relationships with Mencken and Dreiser. One was Fulton Oursler, who publicly admitted to being under Hirshberg's "spell." Oursler testified to Hirshberg's excellent character during the mail fraud trials and, after the physician's sentencing, worked diligently to circulate petitions in both Maryland and New York for the inmate's parole and release. Oursler also kept Hirshberg's name in the newspapers by announcing the physician's active research projects, conducted in prison, on the development of a germ that would kill the boll weevil and on the abnormal psychology of convicted felons. Hirshberg benevolently offered his bogus solution to the South's boll weevil problem to the U.S. Department of Agriculture, "for nothing", but there exists no record of the Department's acceptance of such an offer. Oursler, with the help of many Hirshberg supporters, including motion picture actress Marion Davies (then William Randolph Hearst's mistress), was finally successful in obtaining Hirshberg's parole. The physician-writer was released from the Atlanta Penitentiary on June 24, 1925 after serving only half of his term.

Once out of prison, Hirshberg moved to New York and, on the recommendation of Fulton Oursler, began work with the National Health Service, Inc. Although his title was physician-in-chief, Hirshberg was in charge of writing and editing advertisements for the company. Despite its official sounding name, the National Health Service was fake. Surely Mencken could have written a flaming commentary about Hirshberg's new enterprise. The firm sold useless cures and nostrums through a catalogue entitled *The Book of Health*, including panaceas for pyorrhea, appendicitis, asthma, liver complaints, weakness, mental diseases, and constipation. The catalogue also offered fad foods that "would promote better health," and all were sold with an almost religious fervor by "the world's greatest specialist, Leonard K. Hirshberg, A.B., A.M., M.D. (Johns Hopkins University)." For example, a four-page advertisement in a quack medical magazine called *Psychology* articulated the National Health Service's products and touted Hirshberg in a medicine side-show manner:

> As a forceful, fiery lecturer, he stands pre-eminent. You will hang on his every word—drink in deep his message. As a philosopher, few men have surpassed him. As a medical scientist he is internationally famous. As a consulting physician he enjoys the distinction of having one of the largest practices in all the United States. He is recognized as one of the few great medical geniuses of the present century. You cannot afford to miss this medical scientist's mighty message. He has a pleasing, magnetic personality, a living example of the things he preaches.
>
> Whenever this great dynamic lecturer speaks in public, thousands flock to hear him, vast crowds gather close and strain every nerve to listen. They know his every utterance is of momentous value, that he has something really worthwhile to say. Wise folk, hungry for this new knowledge he is about to impart, will come early at each lecture to make sure of getting a seat, and a FRONT seat at that.[54]

Could Mencken's great hatred for quackery of any kind have been influenced by his acquaintance with the checkered career of Dr. Hirshberg? Certainly Mencken wrote extensively on the theme of quackery with frequent references to its incursions in medicine. He often pontificated about the importance of laughing loudly at quackeries and understanding the jokes of fakery and chicanery.[55] By adopting this cynical but savvy approach to comprehending the world, Mencken reasoned, one would rarely be shocked or disappointed. Yet there exists no record of how Mencken's pen would have captured a real-life quack such as Hirshberg. The final references to Hirshberg in Mencken's 1925 "Autobiographical Notes" and in various letters to friends over the years are somewhat vague and usually relate only to the collaboration on articles and the baby book. In fact, in his "Autobiographical Notes," Mencken makes a point of asserting his lack of contact with the physician:

> Hirshberg later abandoned medicine for various speculations and eventually got into trouble. He is now serving four years in Atlanta Prison. I have not seen him for fifteen years.[56]

As explained by his publisher Alfred A. Knopf, perhaps Mencken was too preoccupied with the "Rotarians, Babbits, and Lower Inhabitants of the Bible Belt" to take an interest in exposing Hirshberg as a quack. It may be that Mencken, well known for his loyalty and fidelity, decided to aim his pointed pen at subjects other than a former friend and collaborator. More likely, Mencken, always aware of his public image as the "Free Lance," probably wanted to avoid public embarrassment and journalistic repercussions and remained rather silent about his relationship with Hirshberg. It was Dr. Morris Fishbein, a frequent contributor to the *American Mercury*, Mencken associate, and editor-in-chief of the *Journal of the American Medical Association*, who publicly exposed Hirshberg's medical activities in 1926. Fishbein accused Hirshberg of being a fee-splitter and a fraud in the *Journal*'s February 13, 1926 issue. Fishbein also documented in detail the less than ethical medical practices of the National Health Service, Inc.[57] Shortly after Fishbein's exposé appeared, Hirshberg's licenses to practice medicine in Maryland, New York, and Vermont were revoked.

Hirshberg drifted from one shifty scheme to another, and although he was never arrested again, it is safe to assume he never truly reformed or settled down to the ethical practice of medicine. Despite numerous scrapes with the law and with medical societies, Hirshberg maintained his innocence or lack of knowledge of any wrongdoing in every single episode. Even in the face of insurmountable evidence, as in the Winthrop Smith blind pool case, Hirshberg would not or could not admit his guilt.

As both a medical reporter for a number of newspapers and periodicals and as popular lecturer, Hirshberg continued to propagate medical fallacies and quack cures well into the late 1940s. Unfortunately, his articles brought letters of desperation from hundreds of ill patients to Dr. Alan Mason Chesney, then Dean of the Johns Hopkins Medical School. Angry letters from physicians protesting the publication of Hirshberg's articles, which advocated resetting the bones of the feet to avoid sciatica and arthritis, the importance of wearing hats to avoid sinusitis, the conversion of bone marrow into a serum called antireticular cytotoxin serum that would fend off cancer, intestinal ulcers, and infections also made their way to Chesney's desk. Chesney patiently but succinctly answered each letter, explaining that Hirshberg had absolutely no connection with the Johns Hopkins Medical Institutions nor did Hopkins in any way endorse his work or writings.[58]

Hirshberg eventually retired and settled down in Long Beach, Long Island, New York. He continued to write and produced a weekly column for the town's local paper called "The Laughable World," took daily swims in the ocean, and, as Fulton Oursler noted, continued to dance with the youngest of girls until he died in relative obscurity in 1969 at the age of 92.

Hirshberg's lasting contribution to American letters, however, had little to do with his own writings; instead, the physician's footnote to posterity was his role in acquainting two literary giants, H.L. Mencken and Theodore Dreiser.

Once the baby book was completed, Dreiser assigned Mencken other writing projects for *The Delineator* and promoted the newspaperman's talents to a number of magazine editors. Mencken encouraged Dreiser to return to novel writing, and, with Mencken's unflagging support as friend, cheerleader, publicist, and editor, Dreiser achieved critical acclaim with such works as *Jennie Gerhardt, The Financier, The Titan,* and, a book that became enormously popular despite Mencken's disdain for it, *An American Tragedy.*

Dreiser's flagrant philandering, obsession with the occult and mysticism, and association with, as Mencken described them, "tenth rate, Greenwich Village geniuses" often exasperated Mencken but the two remained close friends and corresponded daily for a number of years.

Mencken, of course, rose to great fame with his pungent book reviews and literary criticism that advanced realism in American fiction. He subsequently became coeditor (with drama critic George Jean Nathan) of *The Smart Set* and *The American Mercury* magazines. Using these periodicals and his erudite books as platforms, Mencken played a prominent role during the 1920s as the nation's premier commentator on American politics and society, and, as he put it, "disturber of the peace."

Yet despite Mencken's literary success he was to experience difficult times, professionally and personally. Historian T.J. Jackson Lears describes the decline in Mencken's career:

> During the earnestly nationalistic 1930s and 1940s, Mencken's levity seemed an echo of the frivolous Jazz Age. Even during the years of his greatest influence, the 1920s, his ideas betrayed a curiously anachronistic quality. Mencken assaulted Prohibitionists, Rotarians and genteel custodians of culture, but the attack was launched with the well-worn weapons of positivist science and classical liberalism. He clung to the same late Victorian brand of iconoclasm for fifty years, while American culture passed him by.[59]

In addition to his waning popularity with the American public, the death of his wife Sara in 1935 left Mencken bereft and defeated. Nevertheless, he managed to return to the typewriter, perhaps in search of solace, and to produce three splendid volumes of memoirs, *Happy Days, Newspaper Days,* and *Heathen Days,* the fourth edition and two supplements to his magnum opus, *The American Language,* and numerous essays, books, and articles. In 1948 the Sage of Baltimore suffered a devastating stroke that left him unable to read or write and made speaking a difficult task for the remaining eight years of his life. Mencken died in the early morning of January 29, 1956 in the Baltimore rowhouse in which he was born.

Few men were less qualified or less likely to write a book about the care and feeding of babies than the venerable curmudgeon Henry Louis Mencken, yet he accomplished this feat supremely. As Mencken firmly believed, one could learn about and write about anything as long as the appropriate amount of research on the subject was done and professional teachers were avoided at all costs. We can only speculate what Mencken's contributions to pediatrics and the science of childrearing might have been had he stuck to the subject; it seems fortune enough, for both those of us who love children and the prose of H.L. Mencken, that we have *What You Ought to Know About Your Baby.*

Notes

1. Lippmann W. "Book review of HL Mencken's *Notes on Democracy,*" *Saturday Review of Literature,* 11 December 1926.
2. Mencken to Mrs. Helen Dreiser, 30 December 1945, The Theodore Dreiser Collection, Special Collections, Van Pelt Library, University of Pennsylvania, Philadelphia, Pa.
3. Swanberg WA. *Dreiser.* New York: Charles Scribner's Sons, 1956, pp. 119–138.
4. Mencken HL "Review of *Jennie Gerhardt.*" *The Smart Set* 35 (Nov.) 153–55, 1911.
5. Swanberg, *Dreiser,* p. 115.
6. Wilder to Dreiser, 6 June 1907, The Theodore Dreiser Collection, Special Collections, Van Pelt Library, University of Pennsylvania, Philadelphia, Pa.
7. Dreiser T. "Concerning Us All." *Delineator* 70 (Sept.): 284, 1907.
8. Weiss NP. "Mother, the invention of necessity: Dr. Benjamin Spock's *Baby and Child Care.*" *American Quarterly* 29(5): 519–546, 1977.
9. Swanberg, *Dreiser,* p. 122.
10. Washington *Times,* 11 October 1908.
11. Rudolph R. "Aspects of Child Health: Historical Perspectives." In Rudolph AM (ed.). *Pediatrics,* 18th ed. Norwalk, CT: Appleton and Lange, 1987, pp. 1–2.
12. For more information on the Delineator Child Rescue Campaign, refer to *Delineator* magazine: Nov. 1908, pp. 780–782; Apr. 1909, pp. 522, 572; May 1909, pp. 687–689; June 1909, p. 783; Oct. 1909, pp. 300, 352, 384–386.
13. Wilder to Dreiser, 28 November 1908, The Theodore Dreiser Collection, Special Collections, Van Pelt Library, University of Pennsylvania, Philadelphia, Pa.

14. Matthiessen FO. *Theodore Dreiser*. New York: Williams Sloan, 1951, pp. 1106–1107.
15. Mencken HL. *In Defense of Women*. New York: Time Inc. Books, 1963, p. 83.
16. Goldberg I. *The Man Mencken*. New York: Simon & Schuster, 1925, pp. 89–90.
17. Mencken HL. *Newspaper Days*. New York: Alfred A. Knopf, 1941, p. ix.
18. Mencken HL. *Autobiographical Notes* (unpublished manuscript). Henry Louis Mencken Papers, The Enoch Pratt Free Library Collection, Baltimore, Md.
19. Hirshberg LK. Application to the Johns Hopkins Medical School, 20 September 1898, Office of the Dean, The Johns Hopkins University School of Medicine, Baltimore, Md.
20. Oursler F. *Behold This Dreamer!* Boston: Little, Brown, 1964, p. 114.
21. Hirshberg LK. Antitoxin for Hay Fever and Rose Cold. *Maryland State Medical Journal* 67:329–333, 1904.
22. Bode C. *Mencken*. Baltimore: Johns Hopkins University Press, 1986, pp. 145, 248.
23. Hirshberg LK. "Popular Medical Fallacies." *American Magazine* (formerly *Leslie's Monthly* Magazine) 62 (Oct. 1906): 655–660.
24. Hirshberg LK. "Cancer, the Unconquered Plague." *American Magazine* 63 (Feb.): 374–378, 1907.
25. Dreiser to Mencken, 23 Aug. 1907, The Theodore Dreiser Collection, Special Collections, Van Pelt Library, University of Pennsylvania, Philadelphia, Pa.
26. Dreiser to Mencken, 24 Sept. 1907, The Theodore Dreiser Collection, Special Collections, Van Pelt Library, University of Pennsylvania, Philadelphia, Pa.
27. Dreiser T. "H. L. Mencken and Myself." In Goldberg I: *The Man Mencken*. New York: Simon & Schuster, 1925, pp. 378–381.
28. Dreiser to Mencken, 9 March 1908, The Theodore Dreiser Collection, Special Collections, Van Pelt Library, University of Pennsylvania, Philadelphia, Pa.
29. Dreiser, T. "H.L. Mencken and Myself". IN: Goldberg, I. *The Man Mencken*. pp. 378–381.
30. Dreiser to Hirshberg, 6 June 1908, The Theodore Dreiser Collection, Special Collections, Van Pelt Library, University of Pennsylvania, Philadelphia, Pa.
31. Mencken to Dreiser, 16 October 1908, The Theodore Dreiser Collection, Special Collections Van Pelt Library, University of Pennsylvania, Philadelphia, Pa.
32. Mencken to Dreiser, 10 December 1908, The Theodore Dreiser Collection, Special Collections, Van Pelt Library, University of Pennsylvania, Philadelphia, Pa.
33. Park EA, Mason HH. "L. Emmett Holt." *In* Veeder B. *Pediatric Profiles*. St. Louis: C.V. Mosby Co., 1957, pp. 33–60.
34. Holt LE: *The Care and Feeding of Children*. New York: D. Appleton and Co., 1894.
35. Park and Mason, "L. Emmett Holt," pp. 38, 53. See also Randall DA. "Books That Influenced America." *New York Times* Book Review 51:7, 1946.
36. Hubbard ME. *Benjamin Spock, M.D.: The Man and His Work in Historical Perspective*. Ph.D. dissertation, Claremont Graduate School, 1981, pp. 43–49.
37. Ibid., p. 15.
38. Oursler, *Behold This Dreamer!* p. 115.
39. Mencken to Dreiser. Dated "after Feb. 12, 1910." The Theodore Dreiser Collection, Special Collections, Van Pelt Library, University of Pennsylvania, Philadelphia, Pa.
40. See, for example, a series of 3 articles Dreiser published on Madame Eusapia and the supernatural: Rider F. Are the Dead Alive? *Delineator* (Oct. 1908), pp. 539–543, 640–641, (Nov. 1908), pp. 741–745, 849–851, (Dec. 1908), pp. 978–982, 1064–1065.
41. Hirshberg to Dreiser, 4 January 1910, The Theodore Dreiser Collection, Special Collections, Van Pelt Library, University of Pennsylvania, Philadelphia, Pa.
42. Hirshberg LK. The case against Madame Eusapia Palladino. *Med. Pharm Critic and Guide* (NY) 13:163–168, 1910.
43. Dreiser to Mencken, 20 February 1910, The Theodore Dreiser Collection,

Special Collections, Van Pelt Library, University of Pennsylvania, Philadelphia, Pa.

44. Mencken to Dreiser, 27 March 1910, The Theodore Dreiser Collection, Special Collections, Van Pelt Library, University of Pennsylvania, Philadelphia, Pa.

45. Mencken to Dreiser, 10 October 1916. The Theodore Dreiser Collection, Special Collections, Van Pelt Library, University of Pennsylvania, Philadelphia, Pa.

46. Hirshberg LK. Leprosy Now Curable. *Popular Mechanics* 17 (June): 888, 1912.

47. Hirshberg LK. At Last the Cancer Parasite. *Technical World* 18 (Dec.): 399–401, 1912.

48. Hirshberg LK. Bottle Feeding, a cause of bowlegs. *Ladies Home Journal* 37(Apr.):107, 1920.

49. Hirshberg LK. How cancer may be prevented. *Harper's Magazine.* 57 (Mar.): 11, 1913.

50. Hirshberg LK. Menace of eyestrain to the musician. *Musician* 22 (Jan.): 13, 1917.

51. Hirshberg LK. Why a good tenor is sometimes stout. *Musician.* 23 (Mar.): 216–217, 1918.

52. Hirshberg LK. Don the Talking Dog. *Scientific American* 108 (May 31): 502–503, 1913.

53. *Baltimore Sun,* 24 December, 1925.

54. Fishbein M. National Health Service. Capitalizing Ignorance of Diet, Hygiene, and Medical Science. *Journal of the AMA* 86:502–505, 1926.

55. Mencken HL. Preface. *A Mencken Chrestomathy.* New York: Alfred A. Knopf, 1949, p. vii.

56. Mencken HL. Autobiographical Notes (unpublished manuscript), 1925, p. 110 H.L. Mencken Collection, Enoch Pratt Free Library, Baltimore, Md.

57. Fishbein M. *Journal of the AMA* 86:502–505, 1926.

58. Any number of letters in the Leonard K. Hirshberg File, Alan Mason Chesney Medical Archives, Johns Hopkins Medical Institutions, Baltimore, MD substantiate this statement. See, for example letters from Mr. Sterling Moulton of Geneva, Ohio (Dec. 5, 1944), Mrs. Gladys Vicinanzo of Brooklyn, New York (June 2, 1948), Dr. Leon C. Combacter of Fergus Falls, MN (May 11, 1932) as well as Dr. Chesney's responses.

59. Lears TJJ. Ambivalent Victorian: H.L. Mencken. *Wilson Quarterly* Spring 1989.

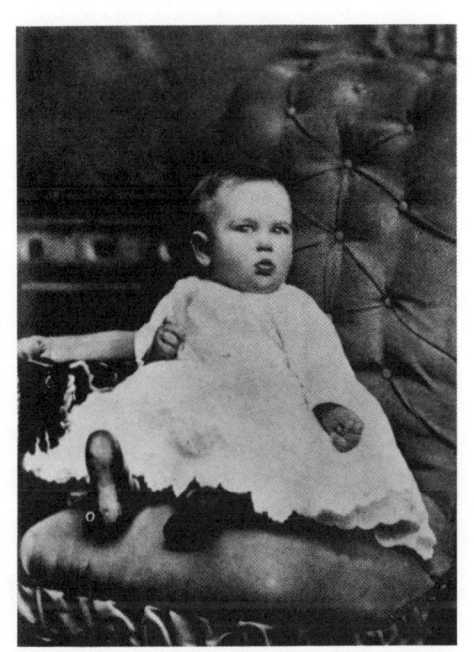

Mencken as a baby. February 1881; W.L. Cover, Baltimore.

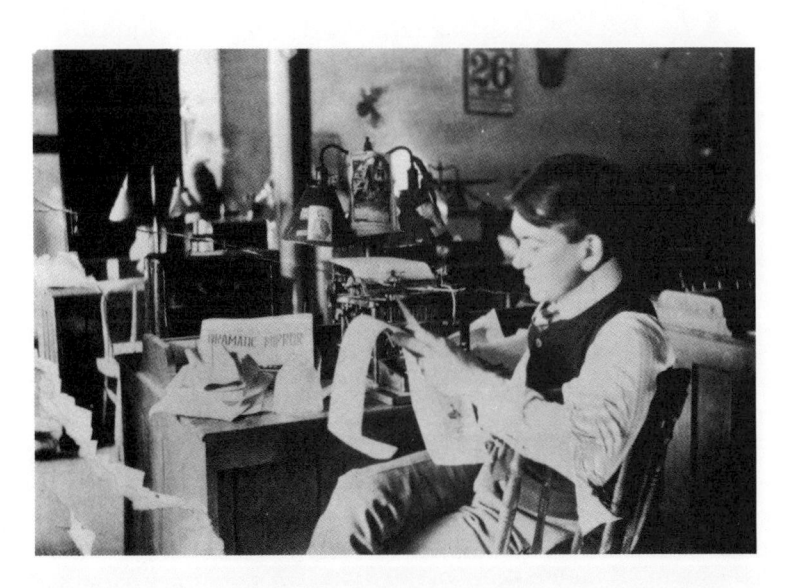

Mencken in the city room of the Baltimore *Herald*. November 1901.

What You Ought To Know About Your Baby

By LEONARD KEENE HIRSHBERG, B.A., M.D.

> *This was written for the Delineator and to the order of Theodore Dreiser, then its editor. I wrote the whole text (save the questions and answers) in collaboration with Hirshberg.*
>
> — Mencken
>
> June 30, 1926

PUBLISHED BY
THE BUTTERICK PUBLISHING COMPANY
BUTTERICK BUILDING   1910   NEW YORK

Inscription in Mencken's hand writing on the title page of the original book in the Enoch Pratt Free Library reads: "This was written for the Delineator and to the order of Theodore Dreiser, then its editor. I wrote the whole text (save the questions and answers) in collaboration with Hirshberg." H.L. Mencken. June 30, 1926.

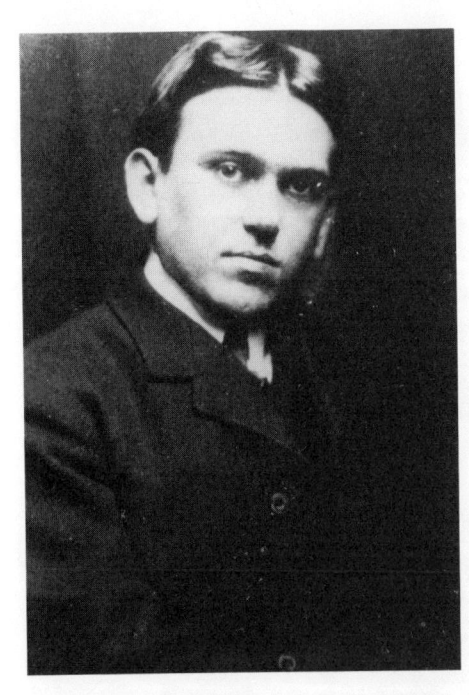

H.L. Mencken at the time of composition of *What You Ought To Know About Your Baby* (1908). (Courtesy of the Enoch Pratt Free Library, Baltimore.)

Theodore Dreiser at the age of 22. (Courtesy of The Theodore Dreiser Collection. Special Collections, Van Pelt Library, University of Pennsylvania, Philadelphia.)

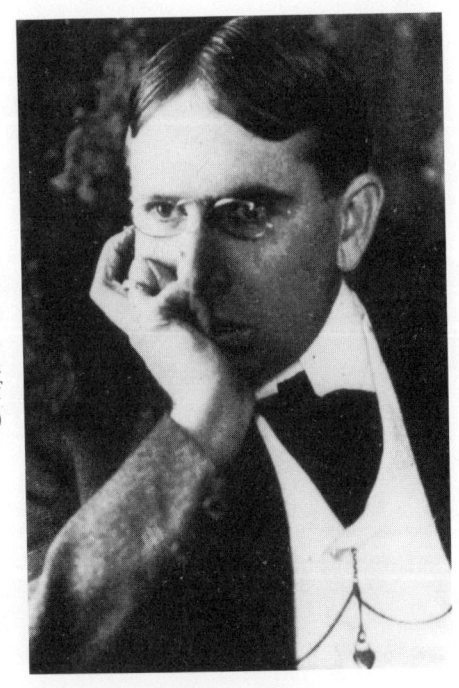

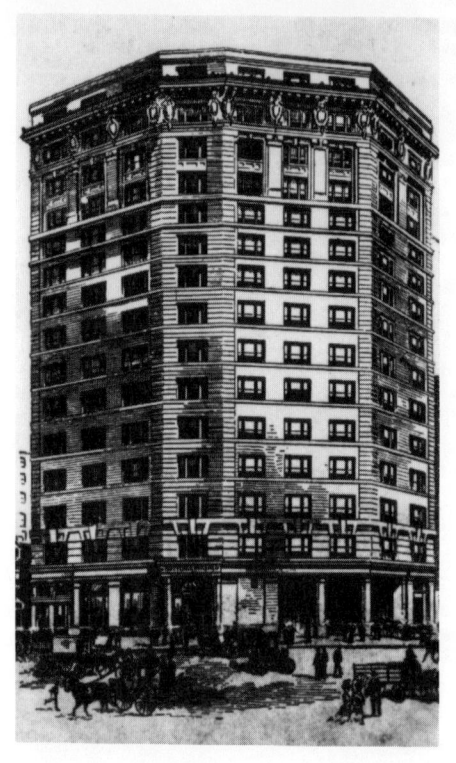

The Butterick Building (c. 1905), a 15-story "skyscraper" on Spring and McDougall Streets in New York City. It is still the headquarters of the Butterick Company. (Courtesy of the Butterick Company Archives, New York.)

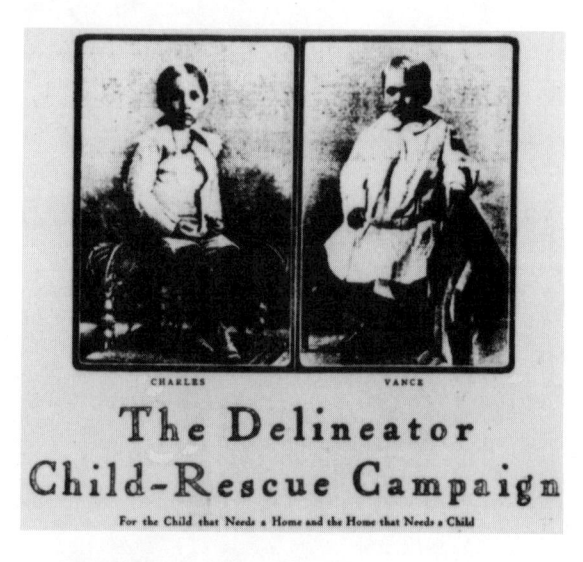

The Delineator's Child Rescue Campaign. (Courtesy of the Butterick Company, New York.)

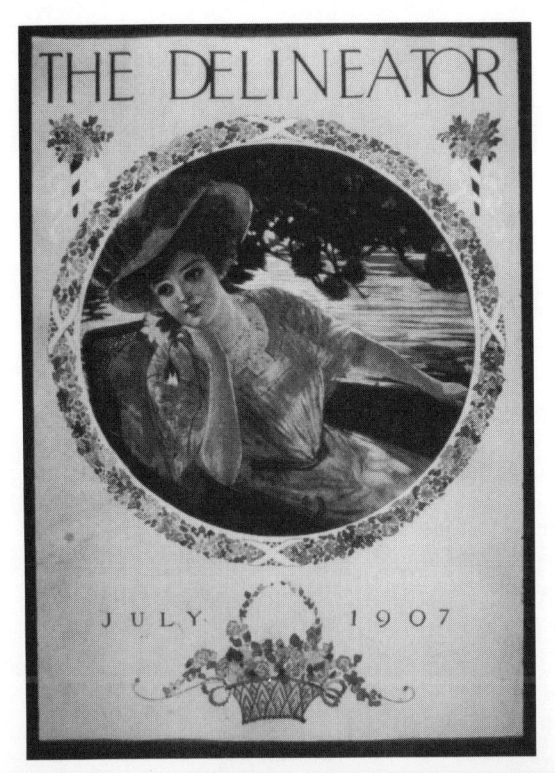

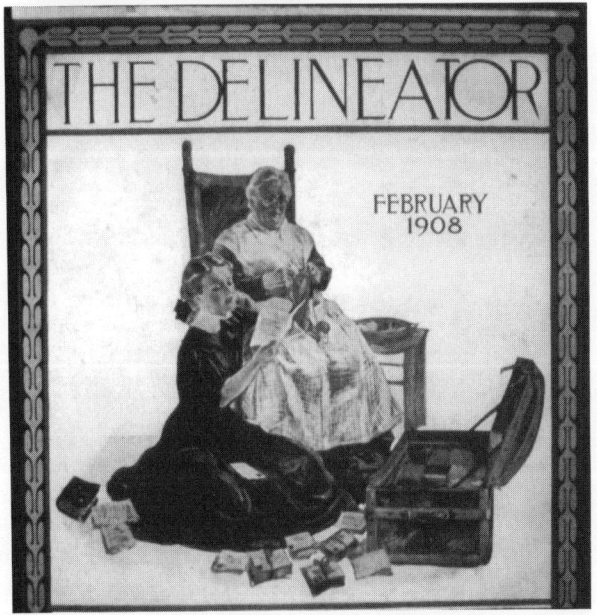

Covers of *The Delineator* from July 1907 and February 1908.

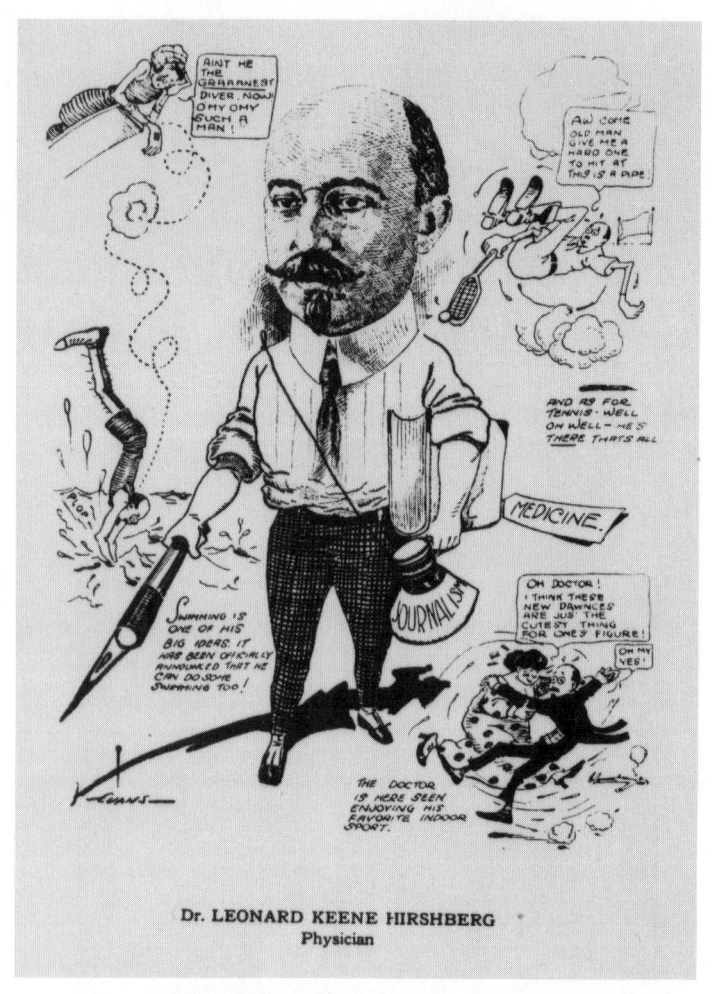

Caricature of Dr. Leonard K. Hirshberg, the physician-journalist who loved to dance with young girls. (From *Club Men of Maryland in Caricature*, Baltimore, 1915, p. 353.)

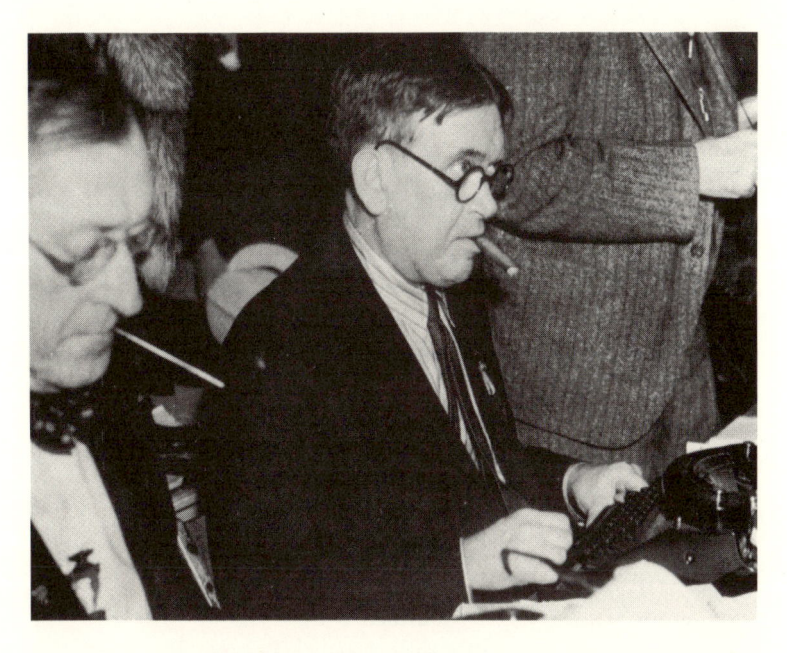

Mencken covering the Republican National Convention in June 1936.

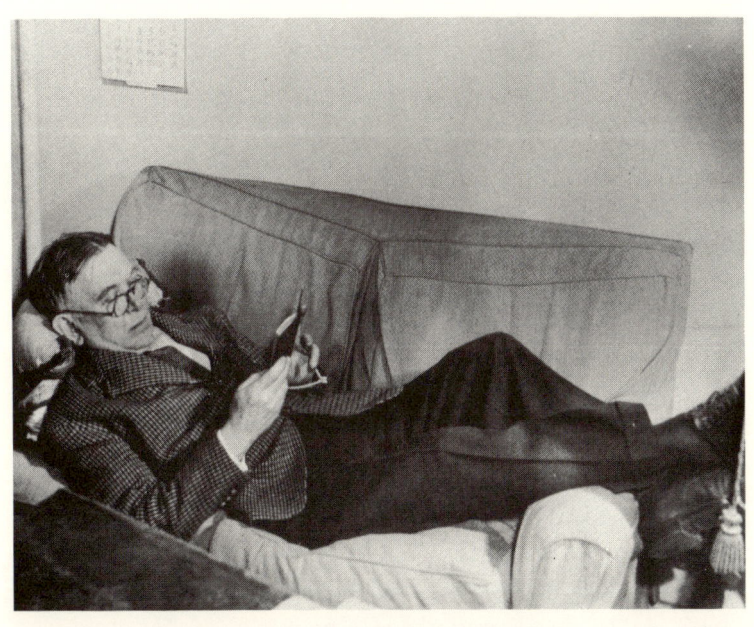

Mencken enjoyed reading in a comfortable position. March 1942; Helen Taylor, New York *Herald Tribune*.

Works of H.L. Mencken

Books

Ventures into Verse (1903)

George Bernard Shaw: His Plays (1905)

The Philosophy of Friedrich Nietzsche (1908)

Men vs the Man: A Correspondence Between R.R. La Monte, Socialist, and H.L. Mencken, Individualist (1910)

Europe After 8:15 (with George Jean Nathan, 1913)

A Book of Burlesques (1916)

A Little Book in C Major (1916)

A Book of Prefaces (1917)

In Defense of Women (1918)

Damn! A Book of Calumny (1918)

The American Language (4 Editions and 2 Supplements)

Prejudices (Series 1 to 6, 1919 to 1927)

The American Credo (1920, with George Jean Nathan)

Notes on Democracy (1926)

Menckeniana: A Schimpflexikon (1928)

Treatise on the Gods (1930)

Making a President (1932)

Treatise on Right and Wrong (1934)

The Sunpapers of Baltimore (1937, with H. Owens, G.W. Johnson, F.R. Kent)

Happy Days (1940)

Newspaper Days (1941)

Heathen Days (1943)

A New Dictionary of Quotations (1942)

Christmas Story (1946)

A Mencken Chrestomathy (1949)

The Bathtub Hoax and Other Blasts and Bravos (1955)

Minority Report: H.L. Mencken's Notebooks (1956)

Plays

The Artist (1912)

Pistols for Two (1917, with George Jean Nathan)*

Heliogabalus (1920, with George Jean Nathan)

*Appeared under the pseudonym Owen Hatteras.

1
The Slaughter of the Innocents

A woman enters a car with a baby in her arms. An old gentleman rises and gives her a seat beside another woman. The baby begins to cry. The mother bounces him up and down.

"I suppose the poor little dear is teething," ventures the stranger affably.

"Yes," replies the mother. "He cut two last week and now he's on his third. It's put him all out of sorts. Last night he had a croupy attack, and if I hadn't given him a dose of ipecac at once we might have had to send for the doctor."

The mother takes a milk bottle from her satchel, carefully wipes the nipple with a rag, and gives it to her offspring. A gurgle—and he is still. The women talk on. The child empties the bottle and begins to fret again. The mother produces a rubber "pacifier" from her capacious hand-bag, and he begins to gnaw it.

"Is he a good child?" asks the stranger. "A real angel," replies the mother proudly. "He never wakes more than twice a night, and then a half-bottle of milk quickly quiets him. My mother has taken complete charge of him. She has raised eight children and knows more than the doctor. She won't let me give him anything but boiled milk."

A common enough conversation, certainly. You have heard it yourself a dozen times, in trolley car and train. It seems utterly harmless—and yet there is in it evidence enough to convict the mother of no less than seven separate and distinct crimes—of omission, commission, ignorance, indulgence and superstition—against her innocent youngster, and, indirectly, against posterity, her country and long-suffering humanity.

Let us go back and listen again. The woman enters the car. The baby begins to cry. She bounces it up and down. Crime number one! Babies should *not* be bounced up and down. It nauseates them; it strains them; it makes them unhappy.

The baby is teething. "It's put him out of sorts." Crime number two!—this time one of superstition. Teething does *not* put a healthy baby "out of sorts." If the little fellow is a normal child his teeth come through the gums without pain. If he cries at the time, the chances are that it is because maternal ignorance has given him bad habits. If that is not true, he is sick, and the chances are that the sickness has its seat, not in his gums, but in his stomach.

"Last night he had a croupy attack, and if I hadn't given him ipecac." Crime number three! For true croup, ipecac is no remedy. For a slight cough—and most mothers group *all* dry coughs under the generic name of "croup"—no medicine is needed. The ipecac makes the little dear vomit; he becomes exhausted and falls into a heavy sleep. Nature cures his cough.

The mother takes a bottle from her hand-bag, wipes the nipple and gives it to her offspring. A gurgle—and he is still. Crime number four! The hand-bag is full of germs, the nipple is full of germs, the rag used to wipe it is full of germs and the bottle is full of germs. Yet the baby lives! And why? Because the human body is so tough that nine times out of ten, in a battle with germs, it wins. But the tenth time it loses.

The child empties the bottle and begins to fret. The mother produces a "pacifier." Crime number five! The "pacifier" is even dirtier than the milk bottle. Germs thrive upon it like barnacles upon a floating log. If the baby is in luck they are the comparatively mild and puny germs, that cause blisters in the mouth, sore gums, stomach-ache, diarrhea and rashes. If fortune frowns upon him, they are the virulent and deadly germs of cholera infantum.

The baby is an angel. "He seldom wakes more than twice a night." Crime number six!—this time one of maternal fondness. A healthy baby should sleep from dusk to dawn without waking. If he doesn't, it is because his mother has permitted him to acquire bad habits.

"My mother has taken charge of him." Crime number seven! True enough, the dear old lady has raised eight of her own. But the acts of her daughter prove that she still clings to a whole confession of ancient delusions. She believes, for instance, that normal teething should torture babies and make them cry. She believes that babies should be nauseated with ipecac whenever they happen to cough. She believes that wiping a rubber nipple with a rag makes it clean. She believes that babies should be bounced up and down, and that, when they cry, they should be given "pacifiers" to gnaw. She believes, in a word, in medical fallacies that were venerable in the days of Hippocrates. And yet she "knows more than the doctor!"

Is the picture overdrawn? Is it a farce? Not at all. Look at it squarely and you will see that it is tragedy—tragedy of the gloomy, every-day sort we have learned to watch unheeding. A hundred thousand American babies die every year. Fully half of these deaths are the sad result, I believe, of unwise feeding, of stupid dosing, of precedent, habit, custom and superstition.

On the face of it, of course, it seems reasonable to maintain that a woman who has brought up eight children of her own, and watched by the bedsides of perhaps a dozen others, should know something about the art. But this conclusion is based upon faulty logic.

The fact that grandma's eight children lived shows only that they were sturdy and lucky—that their natural recuperative powers enabled them to survive her blunders or that they were rescued by some hard-working family doctor. The knowledge that she acquired in raising them consists, in good part, of things that are obviously untrue. Because she once, or twice, or eight times observed that a certain procedure seemed to be followed by a certain result, she maintains, today, as an uncontrovertible proposition, that that same procedure will be followed by the same result inevitably and always.

The doctor is a mere man, and it may be he has no babies of his own, but his knowledge of babies, even accepting the grandmother's test, is infinitely greater than her own. He has walked the hospitals for five years and he has seen and studied, not eight babies, but eight hundred or a thousand. He has read the books; he has listened to the great physicians. He has given his days and nights to the investigation of human maladies—their cause and their cure.

And so, is it not reasonable, when he says that contaminated cow's milk is not good for babies, and that "pacifiers" are likely to inoculate them with the germs of cholera infantum—is it not reasonable to set up his authority against that of the grandmother whose eight babies were lucky and so faced these perils unslain, if not unscathed?

Two considerations must be kept ever in mind in discussing the care of infants. One is the fact that silly superstitions, far from being confined to the slum mothers who give their babies beer and dress them in wadded flannels, are rampant to an astonishing degree among women otherwise intelligent and presumably sane. The other is the fact that the ignorance of the mother, even when the baby passes childhood in apparent health and safety, often paves the way for suffering later on.

The tendency to blame all sorts of things upon intestinal parasites affords a double illustration. A baby, let us say, is restless and fretful. Its body twitches and it moves about in its sleep.

It awakes suddenly and with a frightened cry. By day it squirms in its high chair, picks at its nose and scratches the back of its neck. Its mother is alarmed, and so its grandmother, two aunts and four neighbors are called in consultation. The grandmother has raised eight children; the aunts, between them, have raised nine; and the neighbors point proudly to twenty. Here we have a gigantic conglomeration of expert aid. Thirty-seven human beings are monuments to the science of seven mothers.

"The poor dear has worms," says the grandmother.

"Give him some quassia," says one of the aunts.

"Why not try turpentine?" says the other.

"Or cucumber seeds," suggests one of the neighbors. "When my little Johnnie—"

So the corner druggist makes a sale of shop-worn goods, the child swallows a staggering dose—and during the ensuing forty-eight hours it spends most of its time in a stupor that seems like sleep. Isn't this a proof that it has been cured—by the quassia, the turpentine or whatever other specific the seminary of experts agreed upon? Of course it is!

But all the same a rash intruder might make the observation that babies are not designed by nature for the ingestion of drugs, that a comparatively small dose shocks and exhausts them, and that this exhaustion is often mistaken for healthy and refreshing slumber. And this same observer, sometime later on, might point out that the baby is again wakeful and restless—that it again squirms in its bed and chair and again cries in the night.

In the end, perhaps, it ceases its troubling, and the "cure" is ascribed to the repeated doses that have been forced down its throat. But, on the other hand, there is a chance that it will show no improvement, and that its father, with courage born of alarm, will at last invade the prerogatives of the feminine side of the house and call in a physician. The physician, if all of his honesty has not oozed out of him, will make a thorough examination, and the probability is that he will find the baby to be suffering from adenoids or, perhaps, St. Vitus's dance. [See note on page 44.]

Adenoids are curious little cauliflower-like growths which appear at the juncture of the nasal cavity and the pharynx. They are often observed at birth, but they seldom cause discomfort until some months later. Then they interfere with respiration and cause the baby to be restless. It tosses in its sleep and wakens suddenly, crying out as if in distress.

If adenoids are permitted to remain they deform the mouth, teeth, throat, chest and face. At their worst they produce pop-eyes and what is called a frog-face. They cause mouth-breathing, with all its attendant evils. They open the way for a hundred and one ills, from rupture of the ear-drum, running from the ears, coughs and tonsillitis, to pulmonary tuberculosis.

A slight operation suffices to remove them. The baby suffers little pain and loses little blood. Out they come—and with them the overgrown tonsils that commonly accompany them. If they are suffered to remain, they may never be discovered. But it is certain that in one way or another, they will cause damage.

The mother of eight may say that she never heard of adenoids. But despite her reluctance to include them in her lexicon, they actually do exist. One child in every three has them. In low-lying sea-coast towns they may be found in two children in every three. A generation ago they were unobserved, and it is only for a decade or so that their great importance has been fully realized. And so it is no wonder, perhaps, that the average grandmother is unaware of them. But the poor baby! It pays for her ignorance—in pain, wakeful nights and misery, now and hereafter! Given a child born at full term and of healthy parents, and it is safe to say that half of its infantile ills are due to the ignorance of its mother. She loves it, and so, when it sets up a cry, she nurses it—and it becomes an ill-mannered little glutton, with a penchant for colic. She loves it, and so she feeds it too often and too much—and it becomes ripe for cholera infantum. She loves it, and so, after it has had its fill, she coddles it, bounces it and plays with it—and it vomits.

Despite the general idea that some babies are foreordained to suffer from colic and that nothing can save them, it is nearly always preventable. Its appearance indicates that the little sufferer is getting food of a sort his stomach can't digest, and missing food of the sort he needs. It means that his mother, if he is at the breast, is in no condition properly to feed him. It means that the infant food he is taking, if he is upon the bottle, is poisoning him. The remedy in each case is a consultation with a competent physician. This man, though not a mother himself, will determine exactly what the baby needs, and he will write a prescription that will insure the baby's getting it.

The word "prescription" may suggest the idea of drugs—of paregoric, ipecac, spirits of nitre and all the other ancient contents of the infantile medicine-chest—but in this case the prescription will be, not for drugs, but for milk. What the baby needs is pure, nourishing food, and, failing a good maternal supply, the best food he can possibly get is cow's milk—cow's so modified that it contains the exact amount of proteids, of sugar and of fats that he needs.

In all large cities there are now laboratories, in charge of skilled men, which make a business of supplying cow's milk that has been modified according to physicians' prescriptions. Plain cow's milk is bad for babies, even after it has been boiled, because it lacks certain constituents that they need, and contains others that they should not be called upon to digest. The work of modifying it is done scientifically and cleanly, and the result is the nearest approach to a perfect food that science has yet evolved.

The laboratory man will compound this, and the result will be a bottle of milk—of milk that seems to the feminine expert to be quite like ordinary milk. But when the sick baby has taken it at the hours and intervals laid down by the physician he will have colic no longer, and in the process he will have acquired good habits.

The notion that constant nocturnal bawling is a diversion necessary to the baby's well-being is a fallacy as old as the superstition that sulfur and molasses are good for the blood. If an infant wakes and cries at night it is an evidence of one of two things—either it is ill or it has been permitted to acquire bad habits. If it is ill, the best thing to do is to send for a doctor.

If, after a thorough examination, he decides that it is in good health, the fault lies with its mother. She fed it whenever it cried; she made it associate the act of crying with the production of a meal; she fastened upon it the habit of feeding when it should be asleep.

A healthy infant, properly trained, should go to sleep every night at seven o'clock and sleep soundly until daylight. It should be fed when it awakes in the morning, and it should be fed again at regular intervals throughout the day—every two hours when it is very young, and every three or four hours as it grows older. Its last meal should come just before it is tucked into its crib. And if it cries for food after that, it should be permitted to cry until the habit is broken.

The only things that should ever touch an infant's lips, during its first year, are boiled water and milk—mother's milk, or cow's milk properly modified. If it is born strong and sound and is properly fed it will need no medicines. And all other things—mush, soup, porridge, fruits, pretzels, alcohol, vegetables, meats, "pacifiers," rubber rings, orris-root, sugar, rattles and its nurse's fingers—are abominations in its mouth. They spell indigestion in a dozen forms, not to speak of colic, fevers, wakefulness, faulty growth and cholera infantum.

Next to unwise feeding, as a source of infantile ills, comes overcoddling. Kissing the baby after it has been fed, for instance, is very likely to cause it to vomit, and vomiting is even more exhausting to a child than to an adult. The desire of all aunts, cousins, sisters, grandmothers, neighbors, parlor maids, cooks, seamstresses and other members of the affectionate sex to "hold the baby" and kiss it, and of all uncles, grandfathers and bachelor friends of its father to hoist it to the ceiling, should be rigorously denied. Such delightful domestic pastimes do the baby no good, and very often hurt it. At best it becomes peevish. At worst it shows signs of hysteria. Children should play—when they are old enough to play—with children.

And let there be an end to home doctoring! Most intelligent mothers have learned to be wary of soothing-sirups, but the great majority still put a good deal of faith in paregoric. It is a favorite for diarrhea, stomach-ache and a host of other ills. Often, perhaps, it gives what seems to be relief, since opium, its main constituent, is the greatest of the gifts of the gods. But is it safe for mothers to give their children opium?

In most other home remedies there is less positive danger, but all of them do harm in at least two ways: they postpone the beginning of proper treatment, and they subject the poor baby to excessive and harmful medicating.

Deliberate neglect of her baby is a felony seldom proved against an American mother—or against any mother, for that matter. Yet I sometimes feel that neglect, in the long run, would often do less damage than too much loving. The classical "villainess" of American romance and folklore, who wastes her time in social gaiety and hands over her offspring to professional nurses, seems like some revolting and inhuman monster, and perhaps she is. But did it ever occur to you, oh, indignant critic, that the children of such callous mothers, though they may lack a proper reverence for the canon law and the ordinances against motor speeding, are nevertheless uncommonly healthy animals? The fashionable young woman appears in the divorce courts a bit too often, but she seldom lands in a hospital. She is vigorous and strong. She has a sound digestion. She swings her golf club with muscular arms. And her brother is tough—literally as well as figuratively. He has no morals, but he has a good wind and strong legs.

The cause of all this, I fancy, lies in the fact that these young persons were never coddled. Professional nurses fed them, with inhuman disregard for their yells, upon proper food at proper intervals. An early realization of the futility of bawling led them into regular habits. They swallowed no soothing-sirups; they took no camomile; they knew not the flaxseed poultice nor the home-made liniment. No one rocked them to sleep; no one tickled them; no one bounced them up and down. They were kissed only upon state occasions—and then in a gingerly, aseptic way, upon the forehead or the cheek.

Consider now the baby of the great middle class—the baby enthroned upon a mountain of pillows, the baby whose mother trembles when he cries and worries for days about the mole on his neck and wears herself out slaving for him. How zealously she guards him against drafts! He is clothed in warm flannels; his cradle—he should really sleep in a comfortable crib—is dragged far from the window; he is buried in bedclothes, and he is kept indoors on windy days. The mother's intentions are good, beyond a doubt, but her prophylaxis is hopelessly fatuous. The baby needs air beyond all things. He should spend as much as possible of his first year in the open. He should be taken out in his go-cart upon every fair day, and kept out in all the intervals between meals. He should sleep in a room with open windows, Winter and Summer.

Babies should be put into short clothes at their birth if they come into the world in warm weather, and at two months if they first see the earth in a mantle of snow, and thereafter they should be clad very sparingly.

An infant's skin is so tender that perspiration quickly causes it to chafe. To guard against this the baby should be kept cool and bathed often. And after it has been bathed it should be laid on a clean sheet and not first frescoed with powder and then swathed in habiliments fit only for a mummy.

In Winter the fact that the weather is cold should not condemn the child to hot rooms and bad air. It is easy enough to dress it warmly without burying it in clothes, and if it is warmly dressed the cold will not hurt it. Let it not be understood that I am arguing that infants are fit to face blizzards. But in most parts of the United States blizzards are rare, and the majority of Winter days, though cold, perhaps, are fine. On such days the baby should spend hour after hour outdoors. Awake or dozing, it should be wheeled up and down in the pale sunshine.

The popular notion that all babies are predestined to suffer attacks of a long string of infantile ills, from chicken-pox to diphtheria is utter foolishness. There is no reason, whatever, why a child should take any of these diseases. A baby that has grown accustomed to sunlight and the open—that sleeps soundly, digests normally and has lost, seemingly, all capacity for taking cold—is little likely to fall a victim to the common infections. Its veins are full of good, red blood, and this blood is prepared, at all times, to wage a terrific war upon germs. And even in case the germs prevail, and the baby grows ill, its chance of having but a mild attack and of recovering quickly and without distressing and lingering complications is infinitely greater than that of the vulnerable, ailing, coddled child. The evil effects of coddling do not appear at once. If they did, there would be no coddling. But they appear certainly, none the less, and too often they make the difference between a mild case of scarlet fever and a very bad one, with Bright's disease following after.

The baby that is fed every time it cries, whose stomach is overloaded day and night with improper food, is the baby that falls before the germs of cholera infantum. This is less often a malady of filth—in the popular conception of the word—than a disease bred of faulty nutrition, overbundling and grandmotherly therapeutics. A flaxseed poultice may lay the foundation for pneumonia. A drop of paregoric may kill. A mistaken diagnosis of "worms" may mean St. Vitus's dance, or adenoids and long years of suffering. A flannel garment may pave the way for measles or diphtheria. A home-brewed tea may delay the physician until it is too late. A kiss may spell tuberculosis.

Home dosing and coddling—herein we have the foot-notes that explain the tables of infant mortality. Throw away your paregoric, your ipecac, and your camomile! These things are abominations as bad as your patent soothing-sirups and sarsaparillas. Your baby doesn't need drugs, but pure food and fresh air. If he seems ill, let your doctor prescribe for him. Nine times out of ten he will order milk rather than purges. Open the windows and let in the air! Throw away your stock of chest-protectors, belly-bands and padded woolens! Let the baby kick! Let him breathe! Let him be bare!

Commentary

Chapter 1: The Slaughter of the Innocents

"The Slaughter of the Innocents" was the first article Mencken and Hirshberg wrote for Theodore Dreiser and *The Delineator* magazine. It was submitted in September 1907, although the piece was not published until May 1909. The article is now replete with obsolete ideas but it also offers some excellent advice for mothers even today. The authors introduce two important themes that recur throughout the book. First, they discuss the need for mothers to seek medical advice for their children from trained physicians instead of from self-proclaimed experts such as grandmothers and neighbors. The public's demand for expert opinions on technology, science, and medicine increased during the Progressive Era, and therefore this first theme was largely in tune with the times. Indeed, such demand was the reason for this article. Second, the authors stress the importance of preventive medicine, with emphasis on infectious diseases, the greatest source of infant mortality in the early 1900s.

1. Family remedies and "sirups" Physicians at the turn of the century were strongly influenced by Sir William Osler, the first Professor of Medicine at Johns Hopkins and the most influential physician of the era. Osler was often accused of being a therapeutic nihilist because of his aversion to prescribing many of the commonly used drugs of his day. Osler taught that most of the nonspecific folk remedies and industrial-strength cathartics caused more harm than good. It is not surprising, therefore, that Hirshberg, who walked the wards with Osler as a Hopkins medical student from 1898 to 1902, and Mencken lambaste home remedies such as quassia (bitterwood) and turpentine for the child suspected of having worms; syrup of ipecac, a drug used to induce vomiting and not infrequently given to the child with croup; cucumber seeds, a cathartic that acts much like today's fiber-containing laxatives; paregoric, an opium-containing syrup that slows the movement of the gut and impedes diarrhea; the antiflatulent spirit of nitre; camomile, often infused in tea as an aid to digestion and appetite; and the flaxseed poultice, which was a warm mush of flaxseed contained in a rubber "hot water bottle" and placed on an area of inflammation, either real or perceived, as a means of "counter-irritation."

2. Sleep A brief discussion of the baby's pattern of sleep includes a dismissal of the conventional approaches to getting a baby to sleep that were touted and prescribed in the early 1900s. Mencken and Hirshberg quite rightly identify the leading cause of a baby's irregular sleep pattern as the acquisition of bad habits. Their advice that the baby "be permitted to cry until the habit is broken" was to be echoed 40 years later by Dr. Benjamin Spock:

> Put the baby to bed at a reasonable hour, say goodnight affectionately but firmly, walk out of the room, and don't go back. Most babies...cry furiously for 20 or 30 minutes the first night, and when they see that nothing happens, they suddenly fall asleep.[1]

3. Teething The observation that teething does *not* put a healthy baby out of sorts is still worth heeding. Infants usually begin teething at 6 months of age, starting with the lower central incisors. The teeth generally erupt without event, although local temporary discomfort at the site of a slowly erupting tooth or irritation of gum tissue may occur. Variations in the order of tooth appearance, insufficient space, or dental infections are rarer causes of "painful teething." The approach to teething problems is quite simple. A teething baby who develops irritability, elevated temperature, diarrhea, vomiting, rash, inflamed throat, or other systemic symptoms is ill and requires a doctor's attention, as does the ill baby who is *not* teething.

4. Doctor's advice Mothers are urged to rely upon the counsel of the doctor, who "has given his days and nights to the investigation of human maladies—their cause and their cure." As a physician, Hirshberg obviously had a vested interest in such advice. However, Mencken, too, believed wholeheartedly in expert medical advice and treatment.

QUESTIONS FOR THE MOTHER ABOUT CHAPTER 1

1. Is there anything you would not do to save your baby?

1910 No.

Current No.

2. Is anything too good for your baby?

1910 No.

Current Today's parents need to be wary of the concept of "nothing being too good for one's baby." A recent article by Veronica McNiff in *New York* magazine, "The High Cost of Baby Booming,"[2] estimates that a maternity wardrobe, the medical bills after the insurance company covers 90% of the costs, reading materials on baby care, equipment for breastfeeding, crib, bassinet, nursery supplies, toys, bottles, bibs, utensils, food, pacifiers, teethers, pharmacy supplies, diapers, bathing supplies, clothing, safety measures, pediatric care, and the baby's first birthday party can cost close to $2,200. If you add payment for day care, the expense of moving to a new apartment in order to accommodate the new arrival, and such niceties as a video camera and film to preserve memories of the baby, the cost easily soars over $25,000 for the baby's first year of life!

3. Do you want the best advice in bringing up your baby?

1910 Yes.

Current Yes. Although H.L. Mencken gave people his solicited or unsolicited advice throughout his life, he warned others to be wary of "an idea (a) that is admitted to be true by everyone and (b) that is not true." Nevertheless, good advice is usually a welcome commodity. To parents who seek such advice on the care of their child, we dedicate our efforts.

4. Is grandma's advice or your neighbor's advice the best?

1910 No.

Current The answer to this question probably depends most upon who your neighbors are. Clearly, not all grandmothers or neighbors are qualified to give advice on baby care and it is a good general rule to rely on a physician.

5. To whom can you safely trust your baby?

1910 To the doctor.

Current To a pediatrician, family physician, or qualified pediatric nurse practitioner.

6. Should a mother wait till her baby is sick before taking it to the doctor?

1910 No. The doctor can tell a mother many things about the care of her baby that will keep it from getting sick.

Current No. The importance of prevention as demonstrated by immunizations, anticipatory guidance, and nutritional counseling is even more important today.

7. How often should your doctor see your baby, whether it is well or sick?

1910 At least once in two weeks until two years old.

Current Such strict well-child care emerged in an era when poor nutrition and infectious diseases were the leading causes of illness and death during infancy. As these problems have become less prevalent, the role of the pediatrician has changed markedly, and now includes that of an advisor on behavioral and other modern problems in child care. Currently, the American Academy of Pediatrics recommends 8 to 10 physical examinations during the first 24 months of life or roughly a visit every 3 months. However, studies show a low compliance with these frequency recommendations among all social classes, especially after the first 6 months of life.

8. Is this not an unnecessary extravagance?

1910 No. The cost of a ten minute examination of the baby by the doctor once in two weeks will, in the long run, be very much less than the cost of the doctor's visits and the bills for medicines if the baby has a severe illness.

Current No. Although careful child-health supervision makes logical sense, there exists little clinical data to support the pediatrician's efforts to see children on a frequent basis during the first 2 years. Although such supervision does little to reduce the incidence of acute illnesses, such as infections, a recent study conducted by Dr. Barbara Starfield and associates at the Johns Hopkins School of Public Health and Hygiene came to the following conclusions on the efficacy of well-child care:

> Evidence shows that the frequency of occurrence of conditions that can be prevented declines in response to the provision of medical care; that early detection, when it is appropriate, prevents the progression of conditions from the asymptomatic to the symptomatic states; and that indicated interventions reduce the occurrence of sequelae or prevent the condition from becoming serious. Furthermore, population groups in poorest health appear to benefit the most from improved access to medical care.[3]

9. How many babies die under one year of age in the United States today?

1910 One out of every six babies born dies before it reaches one year of age. One out of every four babies dies before it reaches five years of age.

Current The incidence of infant mortality when Mencken's book was published was closer to 200 deaths per 1,000 live births by age 1 year. The history of Pediatrics as a medical specialty is, indeed, a tribute to modern medicine when one notes the efforts of pediatricians, bacteriologists, immunologists, and public health workers to better comprehend and manage the illnesses cited as leading causes of infant mortality. The mortality rate dropped to 75 deaths per 1,000 live births (7.5%) by 1925 and was 10.9 deaths per 1,000 live births (1.09%) in 1983. Currently, congenital anomalies, prematurity, and sudden infant death syndrome (SIDS) or "crib death" are the leading causes of mortality for babies under the age of 1 year, with infectious disorders such as sepsis and meningitis being comparatively rarer entities. Accidents, particularly those involving automobiles, are the leading cause of death in children 1 to 4 years of age.

11. Shall your baby be the sixth one?

1910 No.

Current No.

12. How can you save it?

1910 By striving to learn the best methods known by experts on feeding, clothing, and caring for the baby.

Current By obtaining good prenatal care from the moment you become pregnant, by avoiding the consumption of alcohol, drugs, and cigarettes during pregnancy, by providing your child with preventive health services including immunizations from a qualified physician, by accident proofing and poison proofing your home, and by feeding the baby human milk during the first 6 months of life.

13. What are some of the superstitions and customs of mothers that make babies sick?

1910 Soothing sirrups; pacifiers; feeding the baby whenever it cries; patent medicines; patent baby foods; family remedies; the idea that babies are doomed to be sick when their teeth come; that the baby must be constantly played with or kept in constant motion; the idea that because so many babies die today they must always die.

Current The belief that infants need medications for every illness, the use of home remedies to treat symptoms of teething, and the belief that infant exercise programs, such as swimming, are helpful to the growing baby.

14. What are the diseases of which babies die?

1910 Diarrhea; pneumonia; whooping cough; tuberculosis; meningitis; and a few of contagious diseases such as diphtheria, measles, and scarlet fever.

Current Diarrhea or cholera infantum was the major cause of infant mortality in the early 1900s before physicians learned to manage it with intravenous fluids and electrolytes in order to prevent dehydration, shock, and death. Unfortunately, diarrhea remains a significant health problem in underdeveloped countries where sterile water and medical supplies are in short supply. It is shocking to note, however, that even in the United States about 500 children per year die from this largely treatable illness.[4] The other diseases mentioned are now treatable or preventable.

15. How many of these diseases are preventable?

1910 All of them.

Current This statement is particularly true today. The typical American infant begins with a safe and effective series of vaccines. Diphtheria, pertussis, tetanus, and poliomyelitis vaccines are administered at 2, 4, 6, and 18 months of age. A booster shot is given at 5 years of age. Measles, mumps, and rubella vaccinations are given at 15 months of age, and a vaccine against *Hemophilus influenzae,* a bacterium that can cause life-threatening infections in the infant, is now available for the child 18 months or older. Most infectious diseases of bacterial origin can be treated with oral antibiotics, easily effecting a cure for otitis media (middle ear infection), pneumonia, "strep throat," and so on. More serious bacterial infections such as meningitis (an infection of the covering of the brain and spinal cord) may require intravenous antibiotics, but these, too, can be well managed by the physician.

16. How many of them are due to ignorance on the part of the mothers?

1910   All of them.

Current   Even the babies of intelligent, caring, and careful parents fall prey to infectious diseases. We do not mean to discount the importance of sound hygienic care for the infant, but for a parent to blame himself or herself for a child's contracting pneumonia, for example, is counterproductive and potentially damaging to the dynamics of the family. The more important message is that if an infant develops fever, irritability, lethargy, diarrhea, vomiting, poor feeding, or other systemic symptoms that seem abnormal, the parent should consult a physician.

17. How many of them are germ diseases?

1910   All of them.

Current   At the turn of the century, all infectious diseases were said to be caused by "germs," in accordance with Louis Pasteur's germ theory of disease. These diseases have long since been classified into specific categories of bacteria or viruses, depending upon the properties of the infectious agent in question.

18. How do germs get into the babies' system?

1910   Through impure milk; through sucking a dirty pacifier or rag; through drinking water that has not been boiled; through nursing bottles and nipples that have not been sterilized.

Current   Germs, or bacteria, have long been known to cause specific infectious diseases in the infant, particularly diarrhea. Bacteria are present in drinking water and milk in minute amounts that usually do not cause disease. They can, however, multiply in unsterilized, unrefrigerated milk or water to the point that drinking such a contaminated formula could easily cause the baby to become ill. Keep in mind that refrigerators were not household commodities until well into the 1920s. Poorly kept milk, usually left on a fire escape or on a melting cake of ice, was a breeding ground for disease-producing bacteria and the leading cause of summer diarrhea. Milk handling during this era was hardly hygienic. Milk was usually transported from the farm to the city retailers' shelves in large 10-gallon cans with little or no refrigeration. At the grocer's, the housewife would dip a portion of the milk from the can into her pail. Bottled milk was not generally available until the 1920s. Because of the ability of germs to multiply, parents are instructed to sterilize formula, nursing equipment, and drinking water before giving them to the baby. Poor handwashing before handling the infant is also an excellent means of spreading infectious diseases.

19. What is the best way to make a baby able to resist germs?

1910 By keeping it out in the air all the time, and by being sure that it is well nourished.

Current The authors' penchant for fresh air finds its origins in a time when many of the readers were city dwellers who lived in less than ideal conditions. The family of 8 to 10 living in a one-room tenement without lavatory facilities, for example, was hardly uncommon. Refrigeration, clean handling of milk, and other important sanitation measures such as efficient sewage and garbage disposal have also been important factors in the better health conditions we enjoy today. Good nutrition, although not discussed in this chapter, is one of the most important factors in the conquest of poor health and disease in this country; it is vital to a child's growth and development. Vaccinations should also be added to the above prescription for fighting infections.

20. Why is the pacifier habit or the habit of sucking the thumb especially bad?

1910 Because it forms the habit of breathing through the mouth. This encourages the growth of adenoids. Because the tissues of the throat become infected with germs taken in this way.

Current The pacifier is often used to prevent thumbsucking and to soothe the "fretful" baby. Approximately 50% of all babies become thumbsuckers in their first 3 months of life. These infants often continue this practice until the age of 3 years or longer. The primary reason for discouraging thumbsucking is its inherent unsightliness, although many physicians and dentists worry about the potential for the thumb to push the baby's teeth out of position ("buck teeth"). As long as the pacifier is washed well between uses, it is a harmless utensil. Most babies will give it up by age 3 to 4 months. Incidentally, the pacifier, thumbsucking, and mouth breathing have no relationship to enlargement of the adenoids.

21. What are adenoids?

1910 Adenoids are small spongy lumps that grow back of the nose and partly close the nostrils.

Current More specifically, adenoids are nodules of lymphoid tissue in the posterior wall of the nasopharynx (i.e., the back of the mouth). Their enlargement can obstruct airflow through the nostrils, causing "mouth breathing," a nasal voice, and snoring during sleep.

22. Why should adenoids be removed?

1910 Because if permitted to remain in the growing child, the mouth, teeth, face and chest become deformed; because they are the direct cause of deafness, constant colds and throat trouble, and often lead to pulmonary tuberculosis.

Current Mencken and Hirshberg derived the concept of enlarged adenoids from the leading pediatrics textbook of the day, *Diseases of Infancy and Children,* by L. Emmett Holt.[5] Holt and other pediatricians were concerned that adenoids and tonsils could enlarge to the point of causing upper airway obstruction with persistent mouth breathing and possible respiratory insufficiency. Deformities of the face (adenoid facies) and chest (pigeon chest) were seen with long-term adenoid enlargement as were frequent attacks of otitis media and possible deafness, nasopharyngitis (infections of the upper airway), and sleep apnea (the brief but recurrent cessation of breathing during sleep which can lead to right-sided heart failure). The authors, based upon information from Holt's textbook, incorrectly attributed a predisposition to pulmonary tuberculosis to enlarged adenoids. Holt also blamed bronchial asthma, urinary incontinence, headaches, chorea (aimless or meaningless movements of voluntary muscles), and epileptiform seizures on the adenoids. Management of enlarged adenoids and tonsils today is based primarily on what they are doing to the patient. They can easily be removed if the child suffers from recurrent infections of the tonsils, adenoids, and throat; if the lymph glands enlarge to the point of obstructing the upper airway or causing apnea (blocking the airflow at the level of the mouth and nostrils for more than 10 seconds despite a child's effort to breathe) or cor pulmonale (right-sided heart failure); or if the child develops an acute abscess of the tonsils or, rarely, the adenoids.

23. How can adenoids be removed?

1910 By a slight surgical operation which can be performed in less than a minute and which causes very little pain, but slight loss of blood.

Current Today, as in 1910, the adenoids can be removed simply and painlessly. The child is anesthetized by a qualified anesthesiologist so that no pain is felt during the procedure. The surgeon removes the tonsils and adenoids carefully with a scoop-like surgical instrument to avoid bleeding. The child then wakes up to one of the greatest ironies of childhood: all the ice cream he can eat and too sore a throat to eat it.

24. Why are mothers glad when they have not delayed in having adenoids removed?

1910 Because the change in the health and happiness of the child is immediate and so marked.

Current Although once the most commonly performed operation in the United States as recently as 1957, pediatricians now send only children who have severe symptoms for a surgical consultation. The most commonly performed operation in children in the U.S. today is the appendectomy.

25. What is the young mother's gospel?

1910 Clean air, clean milk, clean baby.

Current To this we would add time, attention, and involvement as well as a father who helps the mother with all aspects of the child's care. Mencken was to comment upon the importance of husbands helping their wives a decade later in *The Smart Set* magazine article:

> A man makes sacrifices to his wife's desires, not because he greatly enjoys giving up what he wants himself; but because he would enjoy it even less to see her cutting a sour face across the dinner table.[6]

REFERENCES

1. Spock B, Rothenberg MB. *Baby and Child Care*. New York: Pocket Books, 1985, p. 251.
2. McNiff V. The high cost of baby booming. *New York* 18 (July 15):48–54, 1985.
3. Starfield B. *The Effectiveness of Medical Care. Validating Clinical Wisdom*. Baltimore: Johns Hopkins University Press, 1985, p. 145.
4. Ho M-S, et al. Diarrheal deaths in American children. Are they preventable? *Journal of the American Medical Association* 260:3281–3285, 1988.
5. Holt LE. *Diseases of Infancy and Children* (3rd ed.). New York: D. Appleton and Co., 1907, pp. 299–307.
6. Mencken HL. The Altruist. *Smart Set* March 1920, p. 51.

NOTE

St. Vitus's Dance is the chorea, or repetitive, purposeless movements, often seen in a patient with acute rheumatic fever. Physicians originally referred to this form of chorea as St. Vitus's dance in reference to St. Vitus's reputed ability to cure nervous and hysterical illnesses. It is also referred to as Sydenham's chorea after Thomas Sydenham, who provided a superb description of this symptom in his case records of a scarlet fever epidemic during the late 17th century.

2
The New-Born Baby

Just as every man is firmly convinced that he is perfectly competent to drive a nail, run a newspaper or direct the destinies of the nation, so every woman believes that she knows how to care for a baby. The only difference is that the man looks upon his fitness as the result of profound study and a high order of intellect, while the woman, more modest, gives the credit to instinct. Both are wrong.

Instinct and mother love, it is plain, will restrain even the most ignorant young mother from feeding her baby upon cucumbers, but in other ways, unless she is well instructed, she is apt to make mistakes, and these mistakes may be costly. If the instruction she receives comes from one of those well-meaning old women who radiate maternal lore so copiously in all communities, her blunders are certain to be numerous and bad. But if she is sensible, and seeks advice from a physician or a graduate nurse, she will learn a great deal, and the things that she learns will have the merit of being true. With a good groundwork thus laid, she will approach unaccustomed problems and emergencies in an intelligent, efficient fashion.

In choosing the physician who is to assist in bringing her first child into the world, it is well for the young mother to be extremely critical. Unluckily enough, all holders of the doctor's degree are not of the first rank, and very often the man with the most impressive beard and of the most heartening geniality is the least competent.

The best thing to do is to select a practitioner who has been trained in a college of the best sort and who, whether young or old, has standing in his profession. If he is of such admitted competence that his fellow physicians are known to seek and respect his advice, so much the better.

Most towns will have a doctor of hospital experience and skill in conducting infant cases. His fees may seem large, but he well earns them, for his presence is an assurance against many very distressing accidents. The majority of the dangers attending childbirth, indeed, disappear with scientific care. This is especially true of the complications due to infections—childbed fever and blood-poisoning in the mother, and that appalling eye inflammation which leads to blindness in the child. It has been estimated that nearly half of the blindness in the United States today had its origin in infections at birth. A scientific physician knows how to prevent such accidents with almost absolute certainty, but the ordinary neighborhood midwife does not.

The average weight of a white American baby, at birth, is seven and one quarter pounds, but a child may weigh little more than six pounds and still be perfectly healthy. The twelve-pound baby of popular tradition is very rare in fact, and his celebrity is largely due to inaccurate scales and heavy clothes. A child of abnormal size is not to be envied, since he is usually no stronger than a smaller one, and his entry into the world is attended by far greater hazards and difficulties.

A new-born appears such a tiny and distorted caricature of a human being that it is often difficult to convince the alarmed mother that nothing is wrong with it. In color it is a fiery red, and in expression it is utterly vacuous. Its head is large and oblong, and there are spaces between the soft bones of its skull through which the movements of its brain may be observed. The oblong shape of the head soon gives way to rotundity, and the process requires no artificial aid. The notion that the contour of the skull may be modified by the manner in which the child is laid upon its bed has little basis in fact. So long as it is comfortable and has a soft pillow under it, it is safe.

An infant's abdomen appears enormous, just as its chest appears

apparatus has proceeded much further than that of its respiratory organs. For a week or so its breathing may be quick and irregular. Sometimes it will miss a breath, and then again it may breathe so fast that it seems to be suffocating. Do not worry. It is merely a way that new-born babies have.

During its first week the child is apt to lose its red color and become yellowish. Many midwives note this as a dangerous sign, and proceed at once to dose the little one with honey, sulfur and various teas. As a matter of fact, the yellow color is nothing more than the symptom of a passing jaundice which disappears in short order and is by no means alarming. All babies do not have it, but those that do, suffer no damage.

About the same time the child's skin begins to break up into fine scales and come off, and its hair—the fine down on its body and the longer hair which may have covered its head at birth—begins to fall out.

All of this shedding it quite normal, and is a mere preliminary to the appearance of the true, soft, satiny baby skin. With the beautiful texture of the latter every woman is familiar. It is nearly white on the body and limbs, but becomes a deep rose-pink on the palms and soles.

A healthy baby usually celebrates its advent into this wicked world by setting up a shrill cry. When this primal utterance is not heard, the doctor often provokes it by manipulating the newcomer's arms and legs, or even by treating it to a gentle spanking. This cry is a good sign, for it proves that the baby has sturdy lungs and that it has promptly discovered their use. But the absence or postponement of a wail need arouse no fears, for plenty of healthy babies greet the world with dignified silence. It is the firm belief of nearly all midwives that a child which cries feebly or not at all during its first few minutes of life is doomed to illness and early death. This belief is an heirloom from the age of portents and premonitions.

In this connection it may be of interest to note that a new-born baby, no matter how lustily it may signify its discontent, never sheds tears. This is because its lachrymal glands, like many of its lesser organs, have not yet found their function. Neither does it slobber, as babies of larger growth are apt to do, for its salivary glands are still inert, and its tongue, in consequence, is white and dry.

Loving mothers and imaginative aunts are wont to discover evidences of perception and intelligence during the first week, but as a

its acts are automatic reflexes. Crying constitutes the primitive language whereby it makes known its few wants. It cries when it is hungry and when it is uncomfortable. The young mother will quickly grow familiar with its normal voice and so learn to detect variations.

A healthy baby cries about two hours a day for no other reason than that it needs exercise. This crying is not continuous, but is distributed over the twenty-four hours in short spells.

Commentary

Chapter 2: The New-born Baby

The chapter opens with the observation that good parenting skills are not instinctual; they are said to be acquired through diligent, thoughtful care and with the guidance of a competent pediatrician or graduate nurse skilled in pediatrics. Mencken and Hirshberg then turn to the quandary of how to select a competent pediatrician, which is addressed in great detail.

Finding and selecting a qualified pediatrician in 1908 was certainly more difficult than it is today for several reasons. Pediatrics emerged as a specialty separate from internal medicine at the turn of the century. The field at that time was termed "the dependent dwarf of ordinary medical practice" by the eminent medical historian Fielding H. Garrison.[1] There were a few established departments of pediatrics in American medical schools by 1848, most notably Abraham Jacobi's department at New York's College of Physicians and Surgeons. The American Pediatrics Society, one of the first medical specialty organizations in the United States, was founded in 1888. Yet, during the years 1908–1910 there were fewer than 500 physicians in the U.S. who practiced pediatrics exclusively or more than 50% of their time. Finding such a physician outside of the larger metropolitan areas of New York, Boston, or Baltimore was a formidable task and thus an important topic for an article or book on baby care.

Furthermore, any physician who so desired could declare himself a pediatrician and hang out the appropriate shingle without specific training in pediatrics. It was not until 1933 that the American Board of Pediatrics was established and specific standards and qualifications were set upon its examinees. Up until that time it was customary for the physician interested in pediatrics to complete a medical internship at a hospital and then travel to Vienna and Berlin, the meccas of clinical pediatrics, for 2 or 3 months. This brief stint abroad was considered by most physicians and laymen as sufficient training to restrict one's practice to the care of children. Leonard Hirshberg received his "pediatric credentials" in precisely such a manner, spending the summers of 1902 and 1903 observing pediatricians in the "Kinderkliniks" of Berlin and Heidelberg. Not unreasonably, parents had good reason to doubt the expertise of many so-called pediatricians and often felt more confident relying upon the infant's grandmother for health care advice. Mencken and Hirshberg argue strongly against the grandmotherly approach, instructing parents how logically to go about finding a *qualified* pediatrician.

Contrast the paucity in the number of pediatricians in the early part of the century to the quantity of these specialists today. The American

Academy of Pediatrics has over 35,000 members, most of whom are board-certified pediatricians. Board certification means that the practitioner has completed a rigorous three-year internship and residency in a children's hospital and has performed satisfactorily on nationally administered written and oral examinations. These qualified men and increasingly women, who practice throughout the country, must keep abreast of new therapies and current medical management in order to retain their certification by the American Board of Pediatrics. Such a process better insures that parents are consulting qualified health professionals, whose distribution throughout the U.S. makes the location and selection process relatively easy.

Nevertheless, the advice from 1910 on how to select a pediatrician still holds true today. Calling one's local health department or hospital for a list of qualified and highly regarded pediatricians is often a good place to start. Another approach is for the prospective parents to ask friends whose parenting is admirable to suggest a pediatrician. Once a list is generated, it is important to follow through with the selection process by scheduling "prenatal conferences" with the candidates. Such interviews are becoming an increasingly popular way for parents to meet with a pediatrician prior to delivery. During the conference, parents ask questions about the physician's style and philosophy of practice, as well as express specific attributes they seek in a doctor. Some frequently asked questions include information on the fee schedule, whether the doctor is available at nights and weekends, the arrangements for emergency calls if the physician is not available, the physician's qualifications, whether the doctor has specific calling hours, and when the doctor wants to be called about a problem (the answer to the last question is: whenever the parent is worried about a problem he or she cannot handle).

The rest of this chapter touches on several interesting points about the newborn infant that bear some explanation. For example, mention is made of two common infectious disorders that all too frequently accompanied childbirth prior to the antibiotic era, childbed fever and ophthalmia neonatorum.

1. Childbed fever Childbed fever, or blood poisoning (also known as septicemia), is an overwhelming infection of the blood in women who have just delivered a baby. It was first described by Oliver Wendell Holmes, Sr.[2] In 1843, he noted that women who are about to deliver should never be attended by physicians conducting postmortem examinations or examining other women with "childbed fever," lest the disease be carried by the physician from patient to patient. Such a report caused quite a stir among obstetricians, who could not believe they were the cause of so terrible a malady. A study from 1847 to 1849 by the Hungarian physician Ignaz P. Semmelweis confirmed Holmes' statement. Semmelweis found that handwashing with chloride of lime and a nailbrush between deliveries, vaginal examinations, and trips between the bedside and the autopsy suite significantly reduced the incidence of the disease. Such findings were revolutionary in that they predated the acceptance of the germ theory of disease, which stated that agents too small for the eye to see, e.g., bacteria, could cause disease.

2. Ophthalmia neonatorum The "appalling eye inflammation" is caused by gonorrhea and is known as ophthalmia neonatorum, the leading cause of blindness in children at that time. It was usually treated with silver nitrate drops, which eradicated the gonococci but caused a chemical irritation of the eye (conjunctivitis) and swelling of the eyelids. Today, pediatricians routinely instill the antibiotic erythromycin into the newborn's eyes. This drug is better than silver nitrate in that it is less irritating to the eye and it is also effective against another eye infection, chlamydia conjunctivitis, which can be transmitted by the mother to the infant during passage through the birth canal. Chlamydia can also produce a type of pneumonia in newborns, but topical treatment with erythromycin will not prevent it. Prevention can be achieved only by identifying and treating expectant mothers before delivery.

3. The fontanels There are three spaces between the bones of the skull of the infant (called fontanels)—anterior, middle, and posterior—with the anterior being most prominent. The pediatrician is especially interested in the fontanels as the baby develops, because they yield so much information about the development of the skull and brain. The anterior fontanel usually closes anywhere from 4 to 26 months of age, with the average being 7 to 12 months. Delayed closure or a large open anterior fontanel may alert the physician to a diagnosis of hydrocephalus, Down's syndrome, rickets, syphilis, or a large number of genetic and metabolic disorders. An abnormally small fontanel is usually associated with poor brain growth or craniosynostosis, which is premature closure of the sutures of the skull. Finally, the fontanels are a "window" to the infant's brain. One might feel a pulsatile bulge, for example, while the infant cries; such normal "fullness" needs no further investigation. Prominent bulging of the fontanel, however, particularly when the baby is quiet, may be the only hint of meningitis in an otherwise normal infant. Or it may be a sign of hydrocephalus or even intraventicular hemorrhage (bleeding into the brain) in the neonate. Whatever the cause, prominent bulging of the fontanel needs to be examined by the pediatrician. Conversely, a sunken or depressed fontanel can signal severe dehydration and also requires the pediatrician's attention.

4. Hyperbilirubinemia Hyperbilirubinemia, or jaundice, is a yellowish discoloration of the skin that progresses from head to toe. It is caused by an overproduction of a yellow pigment in the blood called bilirubin and an immature liver unable to handle this overload. An elevated bilirubin level in a newborn is a common and generally harmless problem, usually of far more concern to the pediatrician than to the mother and infant. Pediatricians worry about elevated levels because too high a serum bilirubin causes kernicterus, which may lead to profound mental retardation and deafness. This is particularly a concern when the infant's blood type is different from the mother's. Careful analysis by the physician on the timing of the elevation (most newborns have a normal "physiologic" jaundice at age 3 days), the peak level, and the type of bilirubin that is in the blood can usually separate the common, benign, and temporary physiologic jaundice from rarer and more debilitating diseases that can lead to kernicterus. Breastfeeding can also cause a harmless form of jaundice anywhere from 8 days to 2 weeks of life and, in this instance, the therapy is simply to suspend breastfeeding for 24 to 48 hours and follow the decline of the baby's serum bilirubin.

5. Tears and the newborn baby   The authors state that a "newborn baby, no matter how lustily it may signify its discontent, never sheds tears." Actually most term infants do secrete tears. Indeed, the persistent absence of tears is abnormal and can alert the pediatrician to rare disorders of the nervous system. Most infants produce a small amount of saliva at birth and, as is well known to all who take care of children, once the drooling spigot is turned on, it can produce copious fluid on adult shoulders.

QUESTIONS FOR THE MOTHER ABOUT CHAPTER 2

1. Should not the bringing up of a child strong in body and character require a systematic, careful, and scientific study as any profession?

1910   Yes. Enlightened mother-love learns the most advanced methods of caring for children.

Current   Yes. In this day and age of vast communications systems, making information on all topics from baby care to zebra hunting readily available in a variety of styles and formats, it is a simple matter and obligation for contemporary parents to learn about their child's health needs.

2. How can the average mother get this knowledge?

1910   In some large cities and small towns there are classes for young mothers with doctors held in the public schools or in the mothers' clubs. Many health departments send doctors or educational nurses to teach mothers in their homes the care of babies.

Current By asking your doctor for recommended reading material, by obtaining reading information from the public library, or by writing to the American Academy of Pediatrics. (114 Northeast Point Blvd., P.O. Box 927, Elk Grove Village, IL 60009-0927) or the United States Government Children's Bureau (Office of Human Development Services, Department of Health and Human Services, P.O. Box 1182, Washington, D.C. 20013) for pamphlets on child health practices.

3. What should a mother do to belong to such a class?

1910 She should ask her health commissioner or school superintendent whether he can direct her to such a class or send a teacher to her.

Current Unfortunately much-needed classes on parenting are not widely available today. New mothers are often expected to learn skills from reading or attending informal classes held in a pediatrician's office.

4. When should a mother put herself in the care of a doctor?

1910 As soon as she knows a baby is coming to her. She should have a thorough physical examination and should consult her doctor frequently to prevent the dangers that often attend childbirth.

Current Prenatal care should begin once pregnancy is diagnosed. Early prenatal care insures earlier detection of specific risk factors or complications related to the pregnancy. During these prenatal visits, the obstetrician can explain what the mother-to-be should or should not expect during her pregnancy, note what signs and symptoms need to be further investigated, and give advice about diet, rest, exercise, and the avoidance of cigarettes, alcohol, and drugs.

5. Should a mother go to a hospital for her confinement?

1910 If the care of her home and children is heavy, she should do so. The rest and care of the hospital, as well as the education it will give her, is invaluable to her and her baby.

Current Up until the 1930s, it was the practice in this country as well as in other industrialized nations for childbirth to occur at home. Usually the family, with the aid of a midwife, helped the woman in labor. Today, if only as a precautionary measure, a hospital is preferable to the home as a setting for childbirth. In high-risk deliveries, trained professionals in perinatal and neonatal medicine can intervene. In recent years a great many improvements have been made in the physical arrangement of delivery rooms to accommodate the mother and father during the delivery. For example, a supportive companion, usually the child's father, is invited into the delivery room, whereas prior to the 1960s women routinely labored alone. The benefits of this practice have been substantiated by studies showing that more women who had a supportive companion during labor remained awake after delivery and were more interactive with their infants during the time they were awake.

Another innovation is the "birthing suite," a room designed to resemble a bedroom, with minimal interference by the physician or midwife. The birthing suite conveys the sense of delivering at home while still being able to fall back on the resources of the hospital if necessary.

6. What are the tests she should use in selecting her physician?

1910 The best recommendation for a physician is that he is sought by his fellow physicians for advice.

Current While recommendation by another physician is still a very sound criterion, others include: evidence of satisfactory completion of a pediatric residency training program or a family practice residency, certification by the American Board of Pediatrics or the American Board of Family Practice, and satisfaction on the part of other parents who use the physician.

7. What should she do if she is in doubt?

1910 She should go to her health department and ask for advice in selecting the doctor to care for her and her baby.

Current She should call her local County Medical Society or the nearest medical school or hospital-based Department of Pediatrics and ask for advice from the physician in charge of the department.

8. Why should a mother never employ a midwife when she can go to a doctor?

1910 Because many more babies who are brought into the world by midwives die than babies who are brought into the world by physicians. Because a midwife's education falls far below that of a physician. A woman should sacrifice her own prejudice, and always employ a physician. The best is not too good for her baby.

Current Midwives, women who assist in childbirth, have been practicing since at least biblical times, as noted in the Book of Genesis (35:17). In colonial America, midwives were considered important members of the community and continue to remain so in areas where there are few physicians or hospitals. Nevertheless, the reputation of midwives fell drastically by the 1900s, at which time a New York City Health Department study in 1906 stated "over 40% of deliveries were attended by approximately 3,000 incompetent and ignorant midwives."

Although uneducated "lay-midwives" represented an important contribution to the high maternal and infant mortality rates of that time, other factors entered into the picture, such as the practice of women delivering at home instead of in hospitals; the newness of obstetrics as a medical specialty, and its focus on the delivery itself compared with today's emphasis on prenatal, intrapartum, and postpartum care; and the lack of specific state laws and regulations for supervising and licensing midwives. As the 20th century progressed and obstetric care moved out of the house and into hospitals in the 1930s, physicians trained in obstetrics took responsibility for managing pregnancy and deliveries. Midwives who wished to continue their work were required to enroll in special schools.

Today, almost all practicing midwives are "nurse-midwives." These health care professionals are first trained as registered nurses followed by one to two years of study in midwifery and obstetrics. Following such training, the nurse-midwife is certified by the American College of Nurse-Midwives to "manage health care for women without medical problems during the antepartal, intrapartal, postpartal and gynecologic phases of the reproductive cycle, as well as for essentially normal newborns."[4] Nurse-midwives usually practice in a health-care facility where physicians are available for consultation in case of emergency or in the event of complications. In 1982, for example, nurse-midwives conducted 1.8% of the estimated 3,704,000 deliveries that occurred in the United States. Most of these deliveries, 86%, were in hospitals.[5]

The decision to use a nurse-midwife for an uncomplicated delivery, as opposed to an obstetrician who has completed medical school and a four-year residency in obstetrics-gynecology, depends heavily on the philosophies and backgrounds of the parents involved as well as the healthcare resources available. Delivery at home instead of a hospital delivery room or birthing suite is not recommended. If there is the slightest suspicion of a complicated delivery, an obstetrician is strongly recommended.

REFERENCES

1. Abt IA, Garrison FH. *History of Pediatrics*. Philadelphia: W.B. Saunders Co., 1965, p. 130.
2. Holmes OW. The contagiousness of puerperal fever. In *Medical Essays*. Boston: Houghton, Mifflin and Co., 1883, pp. 103–172.

3. Garrison FH. *An Introduction to the History of Medicine*. Philadelphia: W.B. Saunders Co., 1929, pp. 435–437.

4. Varney H. *Nurse Midwifery* (2nd ed.) Boston: Blackwell Scientific Publications, 1987, pp. 3–7.

5. Adams CJ. Nurse-midwifery practice in the United States, 1982. *American Journal of Public Health* 74:1267–1270, 1984.

3
Baby's First Few Months

The young child has almost no power of reason, but, like a little animal, it soon learns to make a sort of unconscious correlation between cause and effect. That is to say, it learns that certain acts lead to certain results. If its nurse or mother stills it once or twice by taking it in her arms, it will cry thereafter whenever it wants to be taken up. In the same way it will learn, in an incredibly short time, how to bring some one to its cradle-side to rock it. These cries of habit should be promptly suppressed, for, in the first place, it is not good for a child to be handled or rocked; and in the second place, compliance will quickly give it perverse and disagreeable habits. Let it cry for three nights in succession and it will hold its peace thereafter. The ancient fear that a baby which is permitted to yell away, without effort to soothe it and still it, will rupture itself, is groundless. A baby lying upon a soft pillow cannot possibly rupture itself, no matter how violently it cries or how vigorously it tosses about.

The cry of habit is much like the normal cry of every baby. The wails are long drawn out and have a sort of rising and falling cadence. They are still at once if the baby gets what it wants. If it does not, they gradually grow less loud and so cease.

The cry of pain, on the contrary, is a short, quick, gasping cry. The baby commonly draws up its legs and gives other evidences of serious disturbance. Mild colic, which is not dangerous, often produces this cry. Unless it is prolonged there is no need to be alarmed. The prudent nurse, however, will make a diligent search for tight napkins and loose pins.

The cry of hunger is a quick, sharp, staccato cry, with high, shrill notes, but less vigorous than the cry of pain. It should cease at once on feeding.

The cry of temper—and temper is exhibited by very young children—is long, sharp, and high-pitched. It indicates that the youngster is enraged—that it wants more light in the room, that its bed is uncomfortable, that it wants some one to change its position, or that it does not want the food forced upon it. Some children have such violent tempers that they throw back their heads and grow blue in the face and seem to cease breathing. The mother often fancies that they are in convulsions and sends for the doctor posthaste. The best way to deal with such recalcitrant little folks is to lay them in bed and let them cry. They will quickly observe the futility of their efforts and so cease.

When children grow older they acquire what might be called the "insulted" cry. A child of six months is sensitive to sharp words and gives voice to the humiliation they produce. This cry consists of a short sob, followed by a longer one, and slowly rising in volume, though not in pitch. Indeed, it is not unlike the cry of a woman.

The cries of pain, hunger and temper are accompanied by a drawing up of the legs. In the other cries the child's limbs have no part.

Babies change so much during their first few weeks that their appearance at birth give no hint as to their future complexion, form or stature. One may come into the world with its mother's blue eyes and small nose, and attain its majority, twenty-one years later with the darker orbs and more formidable nose of its father. This is because nearly all babies have eyes of an indefinite, bluish color, and noses of no particular shape at all. The color of their hair, if they have any, is also misleading, for, as a general thing, it is considerably lighter than it will be in after years.

During its first month a baby has almost no control over its muscles. If you lay it down, it remains just where you put it and cannot change its position. If you hold it up, its head rolls about. In nursing, its movements are entirely automatic and unconscious—as much so, indeed, as those of the minute organisms which bridge the border-line between plants and animals. There is good reason to doubt, indeed, that it is conscious of pain. Its cry appears as a mere reflex and without the interposition of cognition or effort.

But this stage does not last long, for a baby grows with remarkable rapidity. The rate at which it lives is well demonstrated by observing the functioning of its organs. Its heart beats at a rate that would be fatal to an adult, and, as we have seen, it breathes very fast. At birth, for example, its pulse is often one hundred and forty-five a minute, which is just twice the normal rate in a grown man or woman. Its respiration is similarly hurried, being forty-five or more a minute for the first few weeks, as against sixteen to eighteen in the adult. The bowels of a newborn baby are usually very active, but the bladder may not function until after its first day.

By the time it is four months old the child weighs almost twice as much as it did at birth and is plainly making rapid progress. It can now hold up its head without support, and it has developed a habit of grasping any small objects which touch its hands. Before it is a month old it may smile, but it is not until some time later that its smile seems to be associated with any definite idea. By the time it enters upon its fourth month its intelligence is fully dawning. It learns to recognize its mother, and ceases to cry when she takes it in her arms. Its eyes follow lights and moving objects and its ears detect noises.

Soon afterwards it begins to distinguish between its mother and other persons and to become fully conscious of the world about it.

A baby begins to utter sounds other than those of crying when very young, and before it is six months old it often acquires a vocabulary of three or four vowels. The first that it masters is commonly the broad "a," and this diligently repeated, as "ah-ah-ah-ah," convinces its mother that it has learned to say "mama." But, as a matter of fact, the youngster is merely voicing, with the one elementary sound at its command, its general feeling of comfort. This "ah-ah," indeed, is a brother to the purr of the house-cat upon the hearth-rug, and is similarly devoid of any underlying concept.

Soon, however, a multitude of crude but vastly interesting ideas throng the infantile brain, and the baby tries to talk. Some babies make such efforts as early as the ninth month, but others are much slower. The fact that a child is backward in talking is no sign of defective intelligence, nor does it prove that it will be a slow pupil later on. Some of the greatest men of genius the world has known were unable to form intelligible words until the age of two years.

In the matter of walking and teething there is the same unaccountable variation. Some babies are able to sit up at the age of six months and begin to make efforts to crawl at the same time. Held upright on its feet, a youngster of such precocity will try to stand erect, and will crow with delight if it succeeds. There are babies, equally intelligent and healthy, which seem to be hopelessly clumsy and are utterly unable to make the crudest approach to locomotion. As a general thing, a baby which begins to walk at sixteen months is doing well enough. Plenty of children try in vain until after they are two years old. If the baby's legs are strong and it is in good health there is no reason why backwardness in this respect should cause alarm. The various mechanical contrivances for treaching children to walk—rolling chairs, frames, etc.—are of questionable utility and may produce dangerous strains upon the weak bones and muscles.

Commentary

Chapter 3: Baby's First Few Months

"Baby's First Few Months" was written by Mencken and Hirshberg to the specifications of Butterick Publications president George Wilder. Originally appearing in the November 1908 issue of *The Delineator,* the article deals with the baby's pattern of crying and development over the first months of life.

George Wilder, who in 1907 hired Dreiser away from *The Broadway Magazine* to edit *The Delineator* and two other Butterick publications, was a social-minded businessman of the Progressive Era; he was interested in far more than selling copies of magazines or dress patterns. As noted in the introductory chapter, Wilder was deeply concerned about child welfare in America and was extremely supportive of Dreiser's establishing *The Delineator's* Child Rescue Campaigns of 1908 and 1909, a program designed to find suitable homes for orphaned and destitute children. Wilder was also distressed about the alarming infant mortality rate in the United States and hoped that the education of mothers on how to take care of their infants might improve this situation. He therefore pressed Dreiser to publish informative, useful, and understandable articles on baby care for *The Delineator* audience.

1. Crying Wilder's letters and memoranda to Dreiser were quite specific, especially on the topic of crying patterns in infants, which received cursory coverage in the first draft of the chapter:

> It cries when it is hungry and when it is uncomfortable, and the young mother will quickly grow familiar with its normal voice, and so learn to detect variations. If it cries unusually long, or in a strange manner, the doctor is the best person to determine what is the matter.

Wilder wrote Dreiser to ask Mencken and Hirshberg to expand their discussion to include the various types of cries an infant produces and what each type of cry means. For example, "How is the cry of hunger different from the cry caused by pain?" queried Wilder. Wilder learned from Holt's baby book that the average infant cries between 15 and 30 minutes a day simply for "exercise," and felt that this item of interest should be noted. Wilder wanted to include as much information as possible on every subject, in order to provide "sufficient advice... to put the mother wise to a great many things without a doctor." Consequently, he gave Holt's book, *The Care and Feeding of Children,* to Mencken and Hirshberg as assigned reading, and the discussion on infant cries is largely based on Holt's chapter entitled "Cry."

Crying patterns in infants is a subject of current interest to and active research by developmental pediatricians and psychologists. No mere signal of distress, the infant's cry has been found to be a complex vocalization that relays a specific message. One avenue of investigation is the definition of the acoustic characteristics of an infant's cry. For example, specific acoustic characteristics of crying have long been recognized to be associated with Down's syndrome and other chromosomal disorders, hyperbilirubinemia-kernicterus syndrome, meningitis, birth asphyxia, and brain damage. With advances in the measurement of specific components of the infant's cry by using sophisticated tape recording devices and computer analysis, researchers at Brown University and other medical centers are working on means to assess and predict the term and preterm infant's risks for later developmental problems, such as learning disabilities.[3]

Other areas of inquiry in the field of crying include the study of parents' perceptions of the infant's cry and the changes that occur in the infant's crying pattern as it develops. The pediatrician can gain insight into a person's parenting skills by how he or she feels about the baby's crying pattern. For example, a particular cry might signal distress to one parent but bother or annoy the other. Parental responses to crying can influence the infant's overall behavior and its crying pattern. As the infant develops over the first year of life, it will learn to manipulate the vocalizations it has mastered (e.g., crying, babbling, cooing, using specific words) to the situation at hand. The unhappy baby at 8 months is thus better able to express its discontent than the newborn infant. To take this concept further, the angry 2-year-old baby can summon up a virtuoso performance to indicate unhappiness about a particular environment or situation.

2. Developmental milestones The developmental milestones described are still useful for assessing the infant's neurologic progress during the first months of life. An extremely important aid to the pediatrician is written documentation of the date of achievement of each milestone. The parent can record this information in either a prepared "baby book" or in a blank notebook. The list of milestones could easily be constructed from Mencken and Hirshberg's text. For example, did the infant achieve head control by 2 to 3 months of age? Could the baby sit erect at 6 months of age? When did it first crawl? A collection of "developmental notes" facilitates current and retrospective evaluation of the baby's neurologic progress for both parent and physician. Monitoring of milestones is imperative in infants who are at risk for developmental disabilities, such as premature infants, infants with nervous system diseases, or infants with congenital disorders.

3. The tabula rasa "Baby's First Few Months" is an excellent summary of early child development and also shows great foresight by Wilder in its emphasis on the baby's cry. Yet four minor points require clarification. The chapter opens with the statement: "The young child has almost no power of reason, but like a little animal, it soon learns to make a sort of unconscious correlation between cause and effect." The concept of an unthinking infant, the *tabula rasa,* or blank slate, is no longer held to be valid by developmental pediatricians. Dr. T. Berry Brazelton of the Boston Children's Hospital and Harvard Medical School voices the current view of an infant capable of thought:

> There is a zest and vitality in human infancy that shows itself at every turn. The infant looks with absorption, drinks in his environment well before he "knows how" to do anything about taking hold of it. He scouts his world for every sign of what is novel and monitors not only what goes on before him but what is happening at the edges of his world. At the start, in the opening weeks of life, the baby is either alert, "turned on" and in a mood to explore, or he is "turned off" in the total way that young infants have of turning off. Gradually, alertness spreads over longer periods and the infant begins on new tasks—social life, manipulation of things, and the gradual lacing together of the world of the eyes with the world of the hands. A career of self-projected travel begins early—perhaps when the baby can turn from his back to his tummy—and the realm over which control extends expands as no empire ever has.[4]

4. Pain during infancy "There is good reason to doubt, indeed, that it is conscious of pain." In a recent review of the literature on pain and its effects on neonates (babies in their first 28 days of life) by Drs. K.J.S. Anand and P.R. Hickey of the Department of Anesthesia at Harvard Medical School and the Boston Children's Hospital, the incorrect but still widespread belief among physicians that infants do not experience pain is thoughtfully discussed. It is concluded that neural pathways, centers in the brain responsible for the perception of pain, and neurochemical systems thought to be linked to the sensation of pain, are developed and in working order in fetuses and neonates. If one were to measure in a neonate undergoing a painful procedure specific physiologic parameters such as heart rate, blood pressure, respiratory rate, and hormonal and metabolic changes, similar but greater changes are noted when compared with an adult undergoing a similarly painful procedure.[5]

5. Abdominal "rupture" The comment about the baby "rupturing itself" from excessive crying refers to congenital herniations (weak points) of the abdominal wall, either in the inguinal region (groin) or umbilicus (naval). At the time, pediatricians were so concerned about the paucity of fat in an infant's abdominal wall affording poor protection for the organs of digestion that an abdominal "band" of flannel, secured around the baby's belly in truss-like fashion, was often prescribed unnecessarily.

6. Walkers The chapter closes with a comment on walking aids, or "walkers." Although most infants begin to walk at anywhere from 12 to 16 months of age, parents should not be too worried about the otherwise normal toddler who does not walk until 18 or more months. Conversely, some well-developed infants will walk before their first birthday. The authors' reassuring words, "if the baby's legs are strong and it is in good health there is no reason why backwardness in this respect [walking] should cause harm," still ring true. More important, however, is their warning against walkers: "The various mechanical contrivances for teaching children to walk—rolling chairs, frames, etc.—are of questionable utility and may produce dangerous strains upon the weak bones and muscles." This is still excellent advice. When the normal infant is ready to walk, it will. There exists no evidence that walking devices promote early independent walking and, indeed, there is a potential for danger with these aids. One of the greatest dangers of a small infant "wheeling about" in a mechanical walker is that the walker can overturn and the baby, not yet able to cushion the fall, might be hurt. This is particularly true if the infant is playing near a staircase or objects with sharp corners (e.g., furniture). There were over 25,000 "walker-related" injuries, secondary to falls, in the past year alone. Another common but less debilitating problem seen by pediatricians is the mother who comes to the clinic complaining that the baby is holding his feet "pointed out" despite no obvious musculoskeletal abnormality. Invariably this is seen in the baby placed in the type of walker that is most easily manipulated by the baby standing on "tip-toes" and pushing off of them to move. The complaint of the baby pointing out its toes resolves when the walker is returned to its box or a closet and the infant is allowed to continue crawling or cruising until it begins to walk on its own.

QUESTIONS FOR THE MOTHER ABOUT CHAPTER 3

1. What are some of the habits a young baby should be taught to form?

1910 It should be nursed at regular intervals. It should be fed, bathed, dressed, and put to bed at the same hours each day. It should be allowed to sleep most of the day and night except when it is time to be fed or to be bathed. It should be taught to eliminate its food at regular hours. There is no need for the disagreeable and unhealthy custom of soiled diapers. If you hold the child on its little "chair" once an hour, you will help it form clean habits that will prevent constipation.

Current There is no need to establish rigid habits and live life by a clock. The infant should be fed when it appears hungry, which is usually every three to five hours. Although a daily bath is a good idea, there is no need for it to occur at the same time each day. Most importantly, one should not be preoccupied with toilet training during the first year or two of the child's life.

2. Need a baby always wear flannel next to the skin?

1910 A baby should be dressed according to the weather. It should never be allowed to get chilled. It should never be allowed to get into a perspiration, for its body is apt to become chilled. A baby's little body will become chilled or heated quicker than an adult's. Keep its hands and feet warm in winter and dress it very lightly in summer.

Current No. A useful guide to the selection of clothing is the recognition that a term infant, after the first one to two months of life, has temperature control mechanisms similar to those of an adult, so that if an adult would be warm or cold if dressed like the baby, then the baby feels the same way.

3. Should a baby wear long clothes?

1910 If it is born in the cold weather, it may wear long clothes for the first few months, but they must not be long enough to be heavy and drag on the child's shoulders. If it is born in the warm weather, it should wear dresses not below its feet.

Current The length of the clothing is irrelevant except at formal dinner dances. Warmth and comfort should be the criteria by which dress is chosen.

4. What should a mother remember about her baby's clothes?

1910 She should put herself in the baby's place. She should remember that its skin is very tender and that buttons, pins, wrinkles hurt it, make it restless, uncomfortable and fretful.

Current The clothing should be comfortable, made of fire retardant material when possible, non-allergenic, and inexpensive.

REFERENCES

1. Dreiser to Mencken, 16 July 1908, The Theodore Dreiser Collection, Special Collections, Van Pelt Library, University of Pennsylvania, Philadelphia, Pa.
2. Holt LE. *The Care and Feeding of Children*. New York: D. Appleton Co., 1900, pp. 87–89.
3. Lester BM. Developmental outcome prediction from acoustic cry analysis in term and preterm infants. *Pediatrics* 80:529–534, 1987.
4. Brazelton TB. *Infants and Mothers. Differences in Development*. New York: Dell Publishing Co., 1969.
5. Anand KJS, Hickey PR. Pain and its effects on the human neonate and fetus. *New England Journal of Medicine* 317:1321–1329, 1987.

4
The Nursing Baby

A human infant, during the first few months of its life, is an extremely delicate organism, and so it should be handled with care, which means that it should be handled as seldom as possible. The young mother who, in the excess of her pride and love, cuddles her baby to her breast and showers kisses upon it by the half-hour makes a pretty picture, it must be admitted, but it cannot be maintained that the little one is benefited by her caresses. Quite to the contrary, her every kiss helps to make it nervous and irritable and prepares the way for the seeds of disease. A baby that is fondled too much is a baby that cries too much, and is ill too much.

Despite the evidences of intelligence apparent to loving eyes after the first week, an infant's mind is a happy blank, and it gets no joy out of the affections. To it, its mother appears merely as a source of food, and later on, when its brain begins to function, this primitive association of a craving and the means of satisfaction is probably the first definite idea that formulates in its mind. When it is hungry, it wants its mother to feed it, and before long, instead of merely crying for food, it cries for *her*.

When it is not hungry, its chief need and desire is for sleep. A healthy baby, during its first month, should sleep at least eighteen hours a day. And this sleeping should be done, not in a rocking, nerve-racking cradle, but in a solid, comfortable crib. The cradle belongs to the age of spinning-wheels and flails, of soothing syrups and necromancy.

It is not until the fourth day after the baby's birth that its mother's milk is truly nourishing, but such as it is, it exactly meets the needs of the child. It is, in fact, a sort of laxative serum, which stimulates the entire digestive tract and prepares the stomach for the reception of food. On the first day the baby should be nursed only once, but it should be given a drink of boiled water every three hours or so. On the second day it should be nursed three times—morning, afternoon and night—with the same allowance of water. On the third day the routine of the second day should be repeated. At the end of the third day it will be found that the child has lost a quarter or half a pound. This need cause no alarm, for it is perfectly natural, and a steady gain will immediately begin.

On the fourth day both baby and mother are ready for regular feedings at shorter intervals. From this time onward, until toward the end of its second month, the child should be nursed every two hours, with a slightly longer wait after its daily bath, and an interval of seven hours in the night. In all, it should have about nine feedings during the twenty-four hours, as follows: 6, 8 and 10 A.M. and 1, 3, 5, 7, 9 and 11 P.M. Between eleven o'clock in the evening and six in the morning it should not be fed at all. The fact that most babies demand food during this time merely shows that most babies have bad habits. Let the child cry in vain for three nights running and it will never cry again. But during the day, even if it happens to be sound asleep, it is well to waken it in order to keep to this schedule faithfully.

The bath should be given just before the ten o'clock feeding in the morning. The water should be at the temperature of the body—about 99 degrees—and soap should be used very sparingly. After the child has been gently washed, sponge it with a soft cloth dipped in cold water and give it a brief rub-down with alcohol. This will bring the blood to the surface, stimulate the circulation and prevent colds. It is well to let the baby sleep three or four hours after its bath. Then, if it has not already awakened and demanded food, it should be aroused and the regular schedule of feeding resumed.

The length of time that the child should be kept at the breast at each feeding depends so much upon the volume of the milk and its own idiosyncrasies that it is impossible to lay down an invariable rule. The mother should be guided by the fact that a newly-born infant's stomach has a capacity of but one ounce, or eight teaspoonfuls. Some babies are able to ingest this amount of milk in a few minutes, while others require much longer. But it is rarely safe to keep a child at the breast for more than from ten to fifteen minutes.

An infant's stomach is not a fully developed organ, and, as every one knows, it can digest only milk, or something closely approximating milk in composition. As a matter of fact, it probably plays but a minor role even in the digestion of milk, for it stands almost perpendicular and is really little more than an extension of the bowels. The food which enters it passes into the bowels very quickly, and there the more important part of the process of digestion takes place. But, all the same, a baby should be given no more food than its stomach can hold.

A baby, like an adult, needs water as regularly as it needs food. The milk that it gets, though liquid, does not satisfy its thirst. It should be given water at least three times a day, and this water should be nearly, if not quite, free of organisms. The water that comes from the average city main or country spring is alive with microscopic plants and animals, even when it seems clear and sparkling. These minute organisms, as a rule, are harmless to adults, but in the delicate stomach of the baby they are apt to cause disturbances, and so they must be eliminated. The best way to get rid of them is to allow the water to boil twenty minutes. After that, let it cool and store it in clean, well-corked bottles which have been previously immersed in boiling water for five minutes. Glass stoppers are better than corks.

Boiled water is tasteless and insipid because of the absence of air-bubbles, but the baby seldom notices it. It is best drunk out of a thoroughly clean nursing-bottle. Offer water to the infant every four hours, and let it drink as much as it wants. The supply for each day should be boiled in the morning. Under no circumstances should water be kept more than a day.

Commentary

Chapter 4: The Nursing Baby

"The Nursing Baby" addresses four major issues of infant care: "cuddling" or playing with the baby, the baby's pattern of sleep, bathing, and practical advice on breastfeeding. Although subsequent chapters detail the advantages of breastfeeding over formula feeding (please refer to Chapter 5, "Mother and Baby," Chapter 6, "The Bottle

Fed Baby," and Chapter 7, "A Chapter on Milk"), this chapter contains basic instruction on the "nuts and bolts" of breastfeeding.

The chapter begins with strong advice to handle the infant as seldom as possible: " ... her every kiss helps to make it nervous and irritable and prepares the way for the seeds of disease. A baby that is fondled too much is a baby that cries too much, and is ill too much." Although newborn infants require a great deal more attention in their care and feeding than an older infant or child, and while the diseases of the newborn can be far more serious than those seen in older children, such a "hands off" approach is unwarranted. Mencken was so influenced by the concept that newborn infants were "extremely delicate organisms," he later wrote in an article for *The Smart Set*:

> No other animal is so defectively adapted to its environment. The human infant, as it comes into the world, is so puny that if it were neglected for two days running it would infallibly perish, and this congenital infirmity, though more or less concealed later on, persists until death.[1]

Mencken and Hirshberg undoubtedly based their perceptions of the fragility of infancy on the teachings of Dr. L. Emmett Holt. In Holt's book for the general public, *The Care and Feeding of Children*, and in his textbook for physicians, *Diseases of Infancy and Childhood*, kissing the infant is cited as an important mode for the transmission of infectious diseases. In the case of tuberculosis and other airborne infectious agents, such transmission was indeed possible. In an era when no medicines such as antibiotics were available to fight off bacterial infections and modern vaccine therapy was just beginning, doctors had little to offer but strongly worded warnings on disease prevention.

That fondling or playing with the infant is a cause for irritability or disease is unfounded. Infant stimulation provides infinitely more good than harm for the baby's development of personality, intelligence, and the relationship between a parent and baby. The then-popular notion that an "infant's mind is a happy blank, and it gets no joy out of the affections" has been disproved by a host of developmental pediatricians. Paying attention to the baby as it develops and learns new ways to explore its world, and interacting with the baby in a playful manner serve as stimulants to intellectual growth and development.

Mencken and Hirshberg briefly discuss sleeping patterns in infants and are correct that most newborns sleep from feeding to feeding as long as they are satiated and not suffering from any particular problem. Some healthy newborn infants require less sleep than others and their parents have to adapt accordingly. The prejudice against cradles or "rocking the baby" need not be taken to heart. Many a parent and practicing pediatrician swear by the soothing effects of gentle rocking and its uncanny ability to quiet an infant and make him sleepy. The key is *gentle*; remember that rocking an infant is done in preparation for sleep, not as training for a trip to Disneyworld.

The suggestions about breastfeeding are still applicable but need to be amended, especially as they relate to the infant's feeding schedule and its need for supplemental water. Generally, the mother's milk over the first three days of breastfeeding is not milk at all. The fluid produced is called colostrum, and although it is of little nutritional value, it provides the infant with its daily fluid requirements and with the mother's antibodies and immunoglobulins to help the infant fight off infection. As discussed in the subsequent chapters on infant feeding, one of the greatest advantages of breastfeeding is the passage of infection-fighting factors from the mother to the infant. Hundreds of scientific studies corroborate the fact that because of the high content of maternal antibodies in breast milk conferred to infants during feeding (a form of passive immunity), breastfed infants have far fewer infections, both life-threatening and benign, than formula-fed babies.

The schedule of feeding recommended in this chapter should not be taken literally. For example, the baby requires no free water. Although physicians have traditionally suggested 1 to 2 ounces of water once or twice a day between feedings, the amount of water in either breast milk or prepared formulas is sufficient to meet the infant's fluid requirements. During the first 3 to 4 days of life, the infant who is breastfeeding on colostrum will take in enough water to meet its daily fluid needs. One prominent pediatrician has debunked the myth that newborns need water as follows: "If infants were meant to get water, mothers would have three breasts, two to supply milk and one for water." Water fills the baby's stomach but provides no nutrition or calories. There are, of course, certain circumstances when feeding the baby water is a good idea. For example, if the infant has a fever, water might prevent the temperature from rising too rapidly. If the baby is exposed to excessively hot weather, a feeding or two of water between regular feedings will help to prevent dehydration. An excellent way to gauge the infant's needs for fluid is to note how often the baby is urinating or, more simply, to count the number of diapers the baby is wetting; 7 to 8 times per day is normal. The color of the baby's urine is a good indicator of how much fluid is in the infant; dark golden urine or no urine at all are reliable signs of possible dehydration. Incidentally, when feeding the infant water, as with formula, it needs to be sterilized.

The regimented schedule for breastfeeding described is unrealistic and reflects how pediatricians, prior to the Spock era, advocated control of even the smallest details of an infant's daily life. The schedule for breastfeeding depends on more subtle factors than the time of day or night. It is a delicate balance between the infant's level of hunger and the mother's daily schedule.

Usually the breastfed infant indicates hunger by crying loudly every

2 to 3 hours, although a few may wait it out as long as 4 hours. Clearly, breastfed infants need to be fed more frequently than bottlefed ones. A reason for this inconvenience of frequency is that breast milk is the perfect food for infants. As such, it is more easily and efficiently digested than cow milk–based or soy milk formulas, and the baby senses an empty stomach in a shorter period of time. Generally it is best to let the infant nurse for 10 to 15 minutes per side and to alternate breasts for each feeding. The infant gets about 80% of the milk it is going to take each feeding during the first 5 minutes of nursing. Suckling, however, is a soothing, self-regulating activity for the infant, and promotes mother-infant bonding and a sense of well-being. There is an additional bonus in letting the infant nurse for a period of 15 minutes, even if it is no longer taking milk, in that it often calms the infant and helps it drift off to sleep. Contrary to Hirshberg and Mencken's prescribed feeding schedule, a newborn infant should never be left unfed through the night. The infant, especially in the first month or two of life, will not tolerate this and will express its discontent at not being fed for such a length of time. Further, a young infant is at risk for hypoglycemia, or low blood sugar, if left unfed, which can yield a number of complications. The mother should count on at least one to three feedings overnight for the first months of life, depending on the baby's needs.

Another factor that determines breastfeeding schedule is, obviously, the mother herself. The mother's work schedule and type of occupation often play a role in a mother's decision to breastfeed. For example, the filling of the breasts with milk, or engorgement, can be quite painful if left unattended. Mothers often sigh in relief after emptying their breasts, particularly during their first days of breastfeeding. Once the milk begins to flow freely and mother and infant establish a routine, engorgement and subsequent feeding can take place every 2 to 4 hours. Unfortunately, not all jobs allow a woman to breastfeed that frequently during business hours, or the mother may work in an environment where bringing the infant to the workplace for breastfeeding is impractical or impossible. Mothers who are interested in the many advantages of breast milk should, however, be encouraged to use a breast milk pump, which extracts the milk gently. The milk can then

QUESTIONS FOR THE MOTHER ABOUT CHAPTER 4

1. Who should kiss your baby?

1910 Nobody should kiss it on the mouth, not even you. You should instruct every one who is likely to come in contact with it to kiss it on its cheek or forehead. Instruct your nurse not to let strangers kiss the baby. A consumptive's kiss might give it tuberculosis.

Current   Only those who love it, and kissing should not be on the lips except for the mother who is nursing her baby.

2. How much should your baby sleep?

1910   A healthy infant should sleep most of the time except feeding time.

Current   A normal infant, during the first 3 months of life, may sleep from 14 to 20 hours per day. The baby should not be permitted to sleep excessively during the day. If 3 hours have elapsed, the infant should be gently awakened and played with or fed. This will reduce the amount of nighttime wakefulness.

3. Should any attempt be made to develop a young baby's mind?

1910   No. A baby should not even be played with, or in any way excited. This makes it nervous and gives it indigestion. Remember, much joy as your baby gives you, it should never be made to give you, your family, or friends, entertainment at the sacrifice of its own health and regular habits.

Current   Yes. The infant should be spoken to and exposed to music and pictures. Infants are capable of far more observation and learning than we have given them credit for.

4. How should a baby be put to bed in the daytime?

1910   A baby should always sleep alone. It must have a little bed of its own. Not a cradle, but a crib with a flat mattress and a low pillow or no pillow. The baby should be put to sleep on a shaded piazza, or yard, or in a room with the windows open. Its covers should be suited to the temperature of the day. It should never be allowed to become chilled or to perspire. In cold weather the sun should shine on its bed but never in the child's eyes.

Current   The advice from 1910 is still applicable today.

5. What is meant by being "regular" with the baby?

put to sleep at the same hour and taken up at the same hour. That its bowels should move at the same hours – that it should not be fed whenever it cries – not to be taken up to entertain visitors – that it should be expected to sleep all night without feeding or petting.

Current   Being "regular" refers to establishing routines for the baby. Although these patterns are helpful for the mother, there is no scientific evidence that they are necessary for the baby.

6. How often should the baby be bathed?

1910 The baby should be bathed every day before the ten o'clock feeding. Everything necessary to the bath should be in readiness before the baby is undressed. Hang up a list of the necessary articles in the bathroom and consult it every day. The baby may get chilled while you are hunting up something you have forgotten.

List

Tub, warm water, bathroom, thermometer, soap, gauze, cotton wads in covered glass, powder, Vaseline, flannel apron, towel, clean clothes, diaper, alcohol. Solution of boracic acid in covered glass.

Current A daily bath is desirable in the warm weather and once or twice a week in the cold weather. Although no set time for bathing the infant is required, it is vitally important never to use rubbing alcohol to rub down the baby. There have been several cases of alcohol poisoning from rubbing alcohol sponge baths, and the whole procedure is best avoided. Mild soap and warm water are sufficient to clean the baby.

7. How should the bath be given?

1910 Let the room be thoroughly warm before you undress the baby. Be sure there is no cold air on its little body. Wash the baby's eyes and mouth with a swab of aseptic cotton dipped in a weak solution of boracic acid. Wind up a little wad of cotton and clean its ears. Dip a wad of cotton in Vaseline to cleanse its nose. Never stick anything hard into a child's ears or nose, and be careful not to leave any cotton in the ears or nose. A baby's membranes are very easily injured. Then put the child into a tub of warm water and wash it all over with a mild soap. Teach the baby to enjoy the bath. Let it splash about and have fun. It will save you much trouble. Never prolong the bath to please the baby or to entertain friends. Do not let people go in and out of the room while the baby is undressed. Use for a wash rag a piece of aseptic gauze, or bleached cheese cloth, boiled. A sponge catches and develops germs. It is unclean as it cannot be boiled without ruining it. Complete the bath with all dispatch. Wrap the baby in a woolen blanket to absorb the moisture quickly. Powder it with soft powder, dress it and feed it and put it at once to sleep in the air.

Current The baby should be given a daily sponge bath until 2 days after the umbilical cord has fallen off to avoid infections. Bathing should be done using warm tap water and a nondrying soap (such as Dove). The face should always be washed and the eyelids should be rinsed with clean water. The ear canals do not need cleaning. The diaper area should be washed with plain water and mild soap in the male, but soap should not be used in the female to avoid irritating the vagina or the urethra. Never use bubble baths or chemicals in the bath water. When washing and drying the female's diaper area, always wipe from front to back. Make certain the infant is dried thoroughly after the bath. The diaper area may be lightly powdered.

REFERENCE

1. Mencken HL. Man's Place in Nature. *The Smart Set* August 1919, pp. 61–62.

5
Mother and Baby

The nursing-bottle and nipple, whether used for water or for artificial food, should be immersed in boiling water for at least five minutes every day, and when they are not in use they should be kept in a covered glass filled with a weak solution of boracic acid. Such a solution is of constant usefulness in the nursery, and it is well to prepare it in bulk. A cupful of boracic acid, to be had at any drug store, will suffice for two gallons of water. Keep it well covered and it will last for a long while. Use it to wash all dishes, cups, bottles, spoons and other utensils that play a part in the baby's commissariat.

The best possible food for a baby is mother's milk, and this is what it should get whenever possible. The mother who permits social "duties," laziness or any other such excuse or motive to interfere with her highest of privileges is a woman unfit to bring human beings into the world. The best of all infant foods, like the best of all varieties of modified cow's milk, is but a sorry substitute for mother's milk. Nothing devised by the ingenuity of physicians and chemists can so perfectly combine the offices of food, drink and medicine as does this natural food.

When I say medicine, I speak literally, for mother's milk gives to the baby some measure of her own acquired power of resistance to disease. There is, indeed, good ground for the old saying that, so long as a child is at the breast, the blood of its mother continues to flow through its veins. Recent investigation in susceptibility and immunity have shown that this is true, at least in effect, for the breast-fed child shows a distinctly greater capacity for resisting the organisms of all the principal infectious diseases than the child fed upon artificial food. To put it simply, the baby nursed by its mother is far less likely to take measles, scarlet fever or chicken-pox, and far more likely to recover quickly and completely if it does, than the baby nourished by cow's milk and cereals.

Unfortunately, contingencies sometimes arise which make it unwise or impossible for the mother to nurse her child. It may happen, for instance, that the former is suffering from some infectious disease, such as tuberculosis. Under such circumstances, nursing is out of the question, for, besides its dangerous effect upon the health of the mother, it is also apt to bring disaster to the baby.

The child of a consumptive mother should be taken from her at once and brought up away from her. She has a battle for life ahead of her which will consume all of her available energies, and the child, too, has a serious but *not* hopeless battle against inherited predisposition. An infant is ill-fitted to breathe the air of a consumptive's sick-room, and an impulsive kiss may doom it to long suffering—with "spine disease," for example, a frequent form of tuberculosis in children—and an early death.

Any other sort of serious illness is sufficient ground for weaning the child at once. There are also other conditions which make it impossible, however good her intentions, for a mother to nurse her child.

Even while she is nursing her child, some physical or mental disturbance may interfere, temporarily, with a mother's supply of milk. Household cares are often responsible for these difficulties, which show themselves in a scanty supply or in illness in the child. The mother who has half a dozen other children to care for and a house to look after is not capable of providing her baby with the nourishment it needs. During the nursing period she should be relieved as much as possible of domestic cares. Needless to say, she should avoid all excitement of whatever sort. Giving a dinner-party is almost as costly to her strength as a fit of passion or a severe fright, and either may cause the supply of milk to cease or render it unfit for the baby's stomach. Severe intestinal disturbances in nursing children are often caused by maternal imprudences.

The nursing mother should eat plenty of simple, nourishing food, and avoid all stimulants. Alcohol, in particular, is to be held in abomination. She should eat meat sparingly, and should make eggs and vegetables her chief articles of diet. Let her drink milk freely, and avoid coffee and tea. Of raw fruit she had better be wary, but plenty of cooked fruit will help to keep her well. Needless to say, she must pay quick heed to all minor illnesses, particularly disturbances in the digestive tract.

Young mothers are prone to take an unsafe pride in getting about as soon as possible after their babies are born. This ambition, it is plain, deserves no encouragement. The average American woman, especially in the large cities, is far from perfect physically, and so it is well for her to be extremely prudent. But at the end of three weeks it is usually safe for her to take a short drive or shorter walk. As her strength grows she should begin regular daily exercise, preferably walking. Let her keep the windows of her room open, and remain in the open air as much as possible. She needs eight hours of sleep in the twenty-four, at the very least.

When it becomes impossible for a mother to nurse her child, two courses are open: either the baby may be handed over to a wet-nurse, or some effort may be made to nourish it with artificial foods or modified cow's milk.

Wet-nurses, at their best, are unsatisfactory, and at their worst they are exceedingly dangerous. One of them may submit herself to the scrutiny of careful physicians and pass them as perfectly sound, and yet be suffering, all the while, from a communicable malady. Taken as a class, they are ignorant, careless and unclean. Setting aside the occasional gem among them, they seldom provide their charges with nourishment as wholesome as that to be had from the milk laboratory.

Commentary

CHAPTER 5: Mother and Baby

This essay and its companion pieces on infant feedings and the differences between breast milk and cow milk–based formulas ("The Bottle Fed Baby" and "A Chapter on Milk") are the most useful in the text. In an historical sense, it is comforting to know that many of the controversies concerning breastfeeding versus bottlefeeding still exist. Physicians have long proclaimed the importance of breast milk as the perfect food for a growing infant; its easy digestibility, its immunologic properties, and its contribution to mother/infant bonding have all been used as reasons to encourage mothers to breastfeed. Formula manufacturers and many mothers have countered such arguments, from

Mencken and Hirshberg's day to the present, by emphasizing the convenience, easy accessibility, and excellent albeit imperfect nutritional content of commercially prepared infant formulas based on cow or soy milk. This ongoing debate in infant nutrition brings to mind William Shakespeare's words, "What's past is prologue."[1] "Mother and Baby" is still a chapter that any modern-day pediatrician could give to the mother considering breastfeeding, with perhaps a few judicious deletions and additions. The purpose of this commentary is to direct the reader toward the material that is still relevant (e.g., issues on infant infections; the effects of food, drugs, smoking, and alcohol on breast milk; and the mother's mental attitude toward breastfeeding) and away from the outdated topics (e.g., the use of boracic acid as an antiseptic, the risk of tuberculosis from breastfeeding, and the use of "wet nurses").

One passage in "Mother and Baby" exhorting mothers to breastfeed is so pointed and acerbic that it has probably never been equaled in the annals of baby care:

> The best possible food for a baby is mother's milk, and that is what it should get whenever possible. The mother who permits social "duties," laziness or any other such excuse or motive to interfere with her highest of privilege is a woman unfit to bring human beings into the world.

Contrast Mencken's statement to Dr. L. Emmett Holt's more gentle prescription for breastfeeding written at about the same time in his textbook *Diseases of Infancy and Childhood*:

> This is the natural and the ideal method of infant feeding. Every mother should nurse her infant unless there are some weighty reasons to the contrary. The physician should do all in his power to encourage maternal nursing and to promote its success.[2]

Few pediatricians would presume to judge a mother's fitness "to bring human beings into the world" based upon the method she chooses to feed her child, as Mencken bombastically states. Instead, the pediatrician must take Dr. Holt's words to heart. The partnership between a patient and a physician is precisely that, a partnership of two equals, each voicing concerns about a particular decision and, after careful deliberation, reaching a conclusion. Pediatrics is a particularly difficult practice because there exists an added silent, or not so silent, partner—the infant—who cannot yet speak for himself. (We, as pediatricians, argue that the infant would undoubtedly choose the breast.) Nevertheless, there are circumstances in which breastfeeding is not feasible; for example, a mother with cancer undergoing chemotherapy or radiation therapy, syphilis, or tuberculosis; the mother whose breasts do not provide enough milk to sustain the infant's growth; or a premature infant who might have an easier time with other feeding methods. The situation needs to be assessed by the nursing mother and the pediatrician over the course of the first 2 to 4 weeks of the baby's life as mother breastfeeds. One of the easiest methods of measuring the baby's success is to follow the baby's amount and rate of weight gain over this period of time. Usually, a newborn infant loses 5 to 10% of his body weight from water loss during the first few days of life. From then on, the infant usually gains between 1 and 2 pounds per month (approximately an ounce each day) during the first 6 months of life, with a doubling of the birthweight at the end of this period.

The pediatrician should be viewed as a resource for information on breastfeeding and on how to deal with the common problems encountered. The nursing mother needs to be strongly motivated to continue breastfeeding through these first weeks despite potential setbacks such as poor feeding, breast pain, and inconvenience. The rewards on both a medical level, with regard to nutrition, growth, and the prevention of serious infections, and on a personal level, such as the blossoming of mother/infant bonding, are well worth a conscientious and earnest dialogue between the mother and pediatrician.

Today, breastfeeding is enjoying a resurgence in America, particularly among better educated and more affluent mothers. Bottlefeeding, however, remains the principal means of infant nutrition, as it has since its introduction and rapid success at the turn of the century. Dr. L. Emmett Holt lamented in 1907 that breastfeeding was "steadily diminishing" in the United States:

> Among the well-to-do classes in New York and its suburbs, of those who have earnestly and intelligently attempted to nurse, not more than 25% in my experience, have been able to continue satisfactorily for as long as 3 months. An intellectual city mother who is able to nurse her child successfully for the entire year is almost a phenomenon. Among the poorer classes in our cities a marked decline in nursing ability is also seen, although not yet to the same degree as in the higher scales.[3]

Data from the 1970s that were based on the feeding practices of 10,000 mothers revealed that 43% of these mothers left the hospital breastfeeding and 20% of them continued to breastfeed at 5 to 6 months.[4] A similar study of breastfeeding trends from 1971 to 1981 in 51,537 new mothers revealed that mothers who breastfed tended to be more highly educated and have higher incomes, whereas the group that showed the greatest increase in breastfeeding over this time period was women with little or no higher education. It was concluded that good maternal education, prenatally and just after delivery, was instrumental in the rise of breastfeeding among women with little education. Conscientious teaching on the parts of pediatricians and nurse practitioners is probably the key to such an increase. The number of mothers breastfeeding in the hospital enjoyed an annual gain of 8.8%, doubling in size from 1971 to 1981 (from 24.7% of confined mothers to 57.6%). Over the same 10-year period, the number of 2-month-old infants still breastfeeding tripled (from 13.9% to 44.2%).[5] Unfortunately, these and other studies of the late 1970s and early 1980s confirm Holt's 1907 observation that most mothers (75%) stop nursing between 3 and 6 months of the infant's life. Although pediatricians recommend that the longer the mother nurses her baby during the first year of life the better, most would compromise and accept a nursing period of at least 6 months followed by weaning and the introduction of solid foods.

As noted, bottlefeeding became more popular as the 20th century progressed. Although a number of historical and social trends motivated bottlefeeding's popularity and subsequent dominance in infant nutrition, its chief advantage is freedom and convenience for the mother; with the introduction of the bottle, even a father could feed the baby!

Despite trends toward convenience, however, physicians have known from numerous studies conducted over the past 100 years that breastfed infants have a lower incidence of allergies and colic. Most importantly, breastfed infants have fewer infections, ranging from minor infections such as middle ear infections to more serious ones such as meningitis, compared with partially breastfed or exclusively bottlefed infants. Mencken and Hirshberg's aphorism "so long as a child is at breast, the blood of its mother continues to flow through its veins" has been proven correct, time and time again, by the most sophisticated methods of immunology, microbiology, and biochemistry. The nursing mother confers to her infant a number of immunologic factors ranging from antibodies to specific cells that fight off infections. Consequently, breast milk boosts the baby's incompetent and still-developing immune system against the very real threat of an overwhelming bacterial or viral infection. Especially if continued throughout the first 6 or more months of the baby's life, breastfeeding is a natural extension of two other major precautions parents and pediatricians take to prevent serious infections and promote good health in the infant: proper immunizations and supervised health care examinations.

The philosophy that the nursing mother needs to be protected from "physical or mental disturbances" that might "interfere temporarily with a mother's supply of milk" has roots in the tradition of confining a new mother in the hospital for several weeks so that she can spend her time and energy on the newborn infant and nothing else. Physicians still refer to a mother's day of delivery as the "EDC" or "estimated day of confinement. " This protection of the new mother was particularly useful if she had other children at home and the full set of responsibilities that go along with being a homemaker. It enabled the mother to rest and nurse her newborn without worrying about "household cares" or "giving a dinner party." Although the new mother does not need to be confined to her bedroom or the nursery, it remains an excellent idea for the new father to make her transition from pregnancy to motherhood as smooth as possible; this, of course, includes doing the housework! And although a "severe fright" may be contraindicated for new mothers and their babies, an occasional "fit of passion" between parents is usually a welcome activity.

Mencken and Hirshberg note the importance of nursing mothers eating a well-balanced diet and slowly but surely exercising and returning to the pre-pregnant state. Advice is offered on avoiding stimulants, such as caffeine, which can make the baby "jittery," and alcohol during the entire nursing period. Such advice continues to be sound, as does the need for the nursing mother to consult her physician regarding any medications she may be taking. Specific foodstuffs have also been shown to disagree with the nursing infant once they are broken down and secreted into breast milk; the mother who eats chocolate or cabbage while nursing, for example, may cause mild digestive disturbances in the nursing infant.

The American Academy of Pediatrics Committee on Drugs has published a list of medications that: (1) are not compatible with breastfeeding (e.g., amethopterin, bromocriptine, cimetidine, clemastine, cyclophosphamide, ergotamine, gold salts, methimazole, phenindone, and thiouracil), (2) require temporary cessation of breastfeeding (e.g., metronidazole and radiopharmaceuticals), or (3) have caused adverse effects on the infant or lactation (e.g., anesthetics, sedatives including alcohol, specific antiepileptics, antihistamines, decongestants, bronchodilators, antihypertensives, antithyroid drugs, cathartics, anti-infective drugs, diuretics, muscle relaxants, narcotics, and hormones). The list also includes specific foods or environmental agents that might have an adverse effect on the nursing baby, (e.g., aspartame or Nutrasweet, bromides, chocolate, fava beans, lead, methyl mercury, strict vegetarian diets, dry cleaning fluids, and other industrial chemicals).[6] The expectant mother should definitely avoid cigarette smoking, as it has been shown to retard growth of the developing fetus as well as promote birth defects. The nursing mother would be well advised to stop smoking permanently for the sake of her infant's health and her own. The list of harmful agents is quite long and complex and becomes more so each day with the introduction of new drugs and chemicals. The message is that the mother and pediatrician should collaborate on a good drug, dietary, and environmental history to ensure that toxic substances are not being fed to the nursing infant unknowingly.

"Mother and Baby" contains a few statements that are noteworthy for their historical content. The chapter begins with a description of the use of boric or boracic acid as an antiseptic. Boracic acid is a gentle cleaning solution derived from borax and is still available in supermarkets and drug stores. Mothers would prepare a supply in the manner described: "a cupful of boracic acid, to be had at any drug store, will suffice for two gallons of water." Mothers used boracic acid solution to keep the nursery, baby bottles, crib, and other infant-related utensils as clean and germ-free as possible. Although boracic acid works cheaply and well in this role, it needs to be kept out of the reach of other children in the household who might be tempted to drink it. Our present age of disposable diapers, pre-moistened "cleaning wipes," and disposable sterile baby bottles makes the idea of a mother's concocting her own cleaning solution seem prehistoric.

A second important historical point pertains to "the child of a consumptive mother," i.e., the mother with tuberculosis. In Mencken and Hirshberg's day, tuberculosis was an incurable, insidious, and widespread contagious disease. In childhood alone it was one of the leading causes of mortality, claiming the lives of 15% of the children who died in New York City in 1907, for example. The disease was also one of the leading causes of death in this country among people under the age of 50 well into the 1940s. Tuberculosis was rampant among the poorer, malnourished classes, and many physicians incorrectly believed that there was a hereditary component to contracting it. It was, unfortunately, all too common for a woman with tuberculosis to give birth to a baby who was, in turn, at high risk for developing the deadly disease.

Tuberculosis is primarily spread by a person's coughing up infectious material (tubercle bacilli). It is contracted by another person's breathing in this microscopic but infectious matter, which usually locates as a primary focus in the lungs. Tubercle bacilli can be transmitted through breast milk, making even the simple act of feeding an infant dangerous. With such a fear of close contact with persons who had tuberculosis, physicians, unarmed with antibiotics or vaccines, had little choice but to employ quarantine. Many physicians and nurses who specialized in the care of patients with tuberculosis and operated sanitariums had contracted the white plague themselves. Although tuberculosis is now easily cured with a nine-month course of two antibiotics called isoniazid and rifampin, it remains an active infection in the U.S., especially among poor urban dwellers and children. Worldwide, tuberculosis is still a common source of infection and death.

The term "consumption" is an excellent folk name for tuberculosis, in that although it usually begins in the lungs, it eventually "consumes" or infects other organs, including the central nervous system, kidneys, liver, and bones. The "spine disease" mentioned, or Pott's disease, named for the British surgeon Percival Pott who first described it in 1779, is tuberculosis of the vertebrae of the spine. Pott's disease often results in the backbone collapsing upon itself because the bony structures have been rendered weak and incompetent by the dread tubercle bacilli.

Finally, the chapter addresses the archaic custom of wet nursing. Wet nurses were women, usually of the poorer classes, who had recently delivered a baby themselves. Wealthier women, usually those who could not or did not want to breastfeed, hired wet nurses for their infant's nutrition needs. Dr. L. Emmett Holt enumerated the tribulations of wet nursing in *Diseases of Childhood and Infancy*:

> When maternal nursing is impossible or undesirable, the milk of another woman would seem to be the most natural and best substitute. While this is theoretically true, the practical obstacles are so many as to put wet-nursing out of the question as a general method of feeding. We have in America no peasant class like that of Europe to draw upon; and in the class which furnishes most of our wet nurses the capacity to nurse has steadily diminished. The expense of a wet-nurse—twenty to thirty-five dollars a month in New York—the danger of transmitting contagious disease, and the difficulty of obtaining proper care for her own infant, are all very serious objections to wet-nursing.[7]

Dr. Holt's objections to wet nursing in 1907 explains the justifiably brief dismissal of this method of feeding: "Wet-nurses at their best are unsatisfactory, and at their worst they are exceedingly dangerous."

QUESTIONS FOR THE MOTHER ABOUT CHAPTER 5

1. What should a baby be fed?

1910 For the first few months, its mother's milk is the only food that should be given to the baby. The baby should have water three times a day, every four hours, between feedings. It should be boiled and cooled and given in a nursing bottle that has been boiled, or with a spoon.

Current For the first 3 to 4 months of life the infant should be fed mother's milk and nothing more. A nursing infant has no requirement for supplemental water. If breastfeeding is not feasible, then the infant should be fed cow milk–based formula.

2. How can a mother keep her milk in good condition so that it will nourish the baby?

1910 She should eat three plain well-cooked meals a day at regular hours. She should drink water between meals. Keep her bowels regular—constipation in a nursing mother often causes colic in her baby. The baby's health is dependent upon the mother's health. Often when it seems as if the baby must be put on artificial food, by building up the mother's health her milk is improved and the baby thrives on it.

Current The mother should consume an additional 600 calories per day over her regular nutritional needs in order to provide for the increased needs of breastfeeding. The mother should take a supplemental vitamin each day, get out in the sun to increase the vitamin D content of her milk, and consume green, leafy vegetables to increase the vitamin K content of her milk. She should avoid the consumption of whole cow's milk, caffeine-containing beverages, shell-fish, nuts, and chocolate.

3. What may make a mother's milk poor?

1910 Lack of rest and nervousness. Not enough nourishing food. Constipation.

Current Inadequate diet and insufficient rest.

4. What is the mistake most mothers of young babies make?

1910 They try to do too much. They should stay in bed at least three weeks after the birth of a baby, and should cultivate the habit of resting as much as possible before the birth and during the nursing period! It should be a happy, restful time when sleep, food and exercise are abundant. To make it so is the duty of a mother. It is far more important for the future of her family than are the many things she wears out her strength doing.

Current They still try to do too much.

5. Why is nursing so essential to a baby's future health?

1910 Because mother's milk is the natural food. It gives the child the immunity of its parent. It aids the mother by reflexly strengthening her internal organs. A child will grow and thrive on cow's milk, but it has twice as many chances to reach maturity when breastfed.

Current Because it reduces the infant's risk to infection during the first 6 months of life, particularly ear infections, diarrhea, and respiratory infections. Breastfeeding also appears to increase the child's ultimate intelligence quotient (IQ),[8] and to decrease the baby's chances of developing allergies[9] or diabetes.[10]

REFERENCES

1. Shakespeare W. *The Tempest* (act II, scene i). *The Complete Works of William Shakespeare*. New York: Avenel Books, 1975.
2. Holt LE. *Diseases of Infancy and Childhood* (3rd ed.). New York: D. Appleton and Co., 1907, pp. 166–167.

3. Ibid., p. 167.

4. Lawrence RA. *Breastfeeding. A Guide for the Medical Profession* (2nd ed.). St. Louis: C. V. Mosby Co., 1985, pp. 6–21.

5. Martinez GA, Dodd DA. 1981 Milk feeding patterns in the United States during the first 12 months of life. *Pediatrics* 71:166–170, 1983.

6. American Academy of Pediatrics Committee on Drugs: The transfer of drugs and other chemicals into human breast milk. *Pediatrics* 72:375–381, 1983.

7. Holt LE. *Diseases of Infancy and Childhood*, pp. 168–169.

8. Rodgers B. Feeding in infancy and later ability and attainment: a longitudinal study. *Developmental Medicine and Child Neurology* (London) 20:421–426, 1978.

9. Kajosaari M, *et al*. Prophylaxis of atopic disease by six months' total solid food elimination. Evalution of 135 exclusively breastfed infants of atopic families. *Acta Paediatrica Scandinavica* (Stockholm) 72:411–414, 1983.

10. Borch-Johnsen K, Joner G, *et al*. Relation between breastfeeding and incidence of insulin-dependent diabetes mellitus. *Lancet* 2:1083–1086, 1984.

6
The Bottle-Fed Baby

Next to mother's milk, the best of all available foods for human infants is cow's milk. I say "best," but in this connection the word is almost meaningless, for the difference between mother's milk and cow's milk is great. The first is at once a perfect food and an efficient medicine, while the second is a very unsatisfactory food and no medicine at all. That is why a child fed at the breast, all other things being equal, has just about twice as many chances of growing up healthy and sturdy as a child fed from a bottle. Bottle food, no matter how carefully it may be prepared, is a mere substitute and, like all substitutes, it is likely to be dangerous.

The chief superiority of mother's milk lies in the fact that it contains all of the nutritive elements needed by the baby, in precisely the right proportions—*and nothing else*. It is easy enough to prepare an artificial food that contains one or more of these elements, but no man has yet invented one that contains all of them. Again, it is impossible to rid artificial foods of certain things whose presence in the infantile digestive tract causes trouble. Some of these things are merely superfluous, but others are often indistinguishable from poisons.

Saving only the milk sugars and the water, not one of the important constituents of mother's milk is exactly duplicated in cow's milk. Consider, for instance, the difference between the caseins of the two. To understand it, one must remember that a casein is made up of proteids and that proteids constitute the most important of all elements of human nourishment. The albumen found in the white of an egg is a proteid, and the lean part of meat is heavy with proteids.

Well, all proteids, when they reach the stomach, begin to clot, just as the albumen in an egg coagulates when the egg is heated. The proteids in mother's milk and in cow's milk clot in just this way, but what a difference in the manner of their clotting! Those of mother's milk clot into fine flakes, which remain separate and are easily attacked by the secretions of the baby's stomach, and so start at once upon their metamorphosis into blood. But those of cow's milk clot into large, tough lumps, with which the baby's stomach struggles in vain.

The result is that mother's milk is digested easily and rapidly, while cow's milk is digested only with difficulty, and sometimes not at all. This fact explains the frequent colics, vomiting, diarrhea and other forms of indigestion.

Again, cow's milk contains nearly three times as much casein, proportionately, as mother's milk, and in consequence the child who ingests it undiluted is overfed. This helps to burden the harassed stomach and makes the disorder more violent and more frequent.

There are similar differences between all the other constituents of mother's milk and cow's milk, particularly the acids, but they are understandable only to physicians and chemists. More apparent and more important is the fact that cow's milk, as it is received from the dairyman, is alive with a multitude of germs that are never found in mother's milk. There is no doubt that, if the latter were stored in vessels and transported long distances before being fed to babies, it would be just as bad, but every one knows that it is never so stored and transported. It reaches the baby's stomach warm and fresh and without exposure to the air, and so it is always clean and pure.

When a cow is milked the milk takes up floating germs from the air through which it passes in its descent to the can, just as the rain-drops of a Summer shower take up "the gay motes that dance along a sunbeam." These germs, finding the milk a fertile soil, begin to multiply at once and with enormous rapidity. According to some observers, the process begins within thirty seconds. If the can is unclean, or has been washed with contaminated water, if the milkman has dirty hands, or if the cow itself is infected with tuberculosis or any other infectious disease, other and more virulent germs reinforce those of the air, and before long the innocent-appearing can of fresh milk is swarming with organisms.

It is impossible to stamp out these germs entirely, but proper handling of the milk greatly reduces their number. This proper handling looks to two things—a constant low temperature, and absolute cleanliness. The milk must be cooled, and it must be kept cool until it is used. Again, it must be transported, not in open cans, but in air-tight bottles. In practically every American city milk is sold in just such bottles.

Once free of germs, or reasonably so, cow's milk is still unfit to be fed to the baby, for its proteids, sugar, fats and acids are yet present in improper proportions. It has, for instance, certain strange acids, and these must be neutralized.

I desire to impress upon all mothers, the desirability of seeking advice from a good physician whenever it becomes necessary to take the baby from the breast. Only a doctor can accurately determine the needs of a given child.

In most cities there are milk laboratories which make a business of modifying cow's milk upon prescription. The physician, knowing the child's peculiar requirements, decides just how much casein, sugar and fats should enter into each quart of milk that it ingests, and the laboratory prepares a milk containing these things in exactly the right proportions. Such milk may be prepared at home by the mother under a physician's direction.

Until it is six months old the bottle-fed baby should take nothing but modified milk and boiled water into its stomach. It should be fed according to the schedule I have laid down for breast-fed children, and should get just as much water. The strength of the modified milk should be increased from month to month. During the first few weeks it may be advisable to use four, five or even six parts of water to one of milk, but after the first month the proportion of milk may be increased in amount quite rapidly. By the end of the second month, if the baby seems to be thriving, it may take equal parts of milk and water, and later on the milk may exceed the water until, toward the end of the first year, the child may take almost pure milk. But this should be managed with caution, and at the first sign of digestive disturbance there should be a wise retreat.

When the first teeth appear it is time to add something more substantial to the diet. Many physicians condemn baby foods without reservation, but in this I cannot concur. Wisely employed, they are often of great value, but it is not wise to use them unless absolutely necessary, and then only in selected instances. I often, but not always, add them cautiously to the milk, beginning with very little milk, then, if all goes well, gradually increase the proportion. Such foods should not be used save in such conjunction with milk. In selecting a food it is well to remember that the advice of your doctor is far more valuable than that of your neighbor, for babies differ.

By the time the baby is a year old its diet should begin to include fruit juices and the whites of eggs. Begin with a wine-glass of chicken broth or bouillon, fed from a spoon, and as these things are increased, gradually decrease the amount of bottle food. Soon after it turns its first year the child should learn to drink from a small cup. After that its meals may be reduced to five a day, with an occasional drink of orange juice and plenty of water.

The first meal should have modified milk as its chief constituent, with half as much infant food or strained oatmeal added. The second meal, in the middle of the morning, may be a repetition of the first. Early in the afternoon a gill of chicken broth, or half as much beef juice, may be given, and this may be varied every few days, with the white of an egg boiled, say, for a minute. The two remaining meals should have milk as their mainstay. After a month or so of such diet, if the baby is in good health, its mid-morning meal may begin to include dry toast, zwieback, thin oatmeal and other cereals, and its afternoon dinner may include a whole egg, soft-boiled or poached. Fruits should be given freely, but it is always best to have them well cooked.

I need scarcely refer again to the need for keeping all bottles, nipples, glasses and spoons absolutely clean. They should be scalded after every meal, and should be kept, between meals, in a vessel filled with a dilute solution of boracic acid. Just before using they should be washed thoroughly in very hot water. Particular attention must be paid to the rubber nipples. They are veritable havens for wandering germs.

7
A Chapter on Milk

After all, those socialists who insist that the bread-and-butter problem is the one all-inclusive human problem are not very far from right. A man's mental, moral and physical make-up depends, to a degree incredible to the casual observer, upon the food he eats, and, to a degree still more incredible, upon the food he ate when he was a baby. Save only the air he breathes, nothing more potently determines the sort of man he is to be—not even his nationality or his faith.

Of course, it is impossible to find out, with any approach to exactness, the eventual effect of a given foodstuff, but every one is well aware of the peculiar emotional consequences which arise out of certain general conditions of diet. The starving man has no conscience, and the dyspeptic has no soul. At the other pole stands the well-fed man of sound stomach. He is as happy after dinner as any human being can ever hope to be.

Between these two extremes one may find a thousand other proofs, physical and psychological, of the effect of food upon the human animal. It is, indeed, fast becoming a favorite theory among biologists that many of those changes which cause the evolution of species are due to changes in nutrition; and there is even some ground for believing that man's enormous superiority over all other beings to-day is due in part to the fact that his remote ancestors, one lucky day, discovered the art of cookery.

Nature provides the best of all possible foods for babies in mother's milk, but accidents often make this unavailable, and so it becomes necessary to seek a substitute. This substitute has almost invariably been the milk of the cow, the goat, the reindeer, the horse or the camel. Until recently it was generally believed that the substitute was as good as the thing it supplanted. But one day there appeared a man named Louis Pasteur, who showed the world that cow's milk, to name but one of these substitutes, was always a dangerous food, and that, in a great many cases, it was a violent and fatal poison.

Pasteur proved this by his discovery that cow's milk, by the time it reaches the nursery, always contains microscopic forms of life. Some of these minute organisms, pehaps, are harmless enough, but others are the very reverse. So noxious are they, in fact, that it is fair to blame them for a large proportion of the maladies of childhood, and, in addition, for not a few of those defects of bodily function which, while not at once fatal, pave the way for illness and death later on—perhaps as late as middle life.

The layman may here want to know why it is that cow's milk, if it is so badly contaminated, does not poison the calves for whom nature intended it; and why, again, if cow's milk is so dangerous, mother's milk is not just as bad. The answer lies in the fact that, when any milk is fed to the offspring of its mother in the way nature intended it to be fed, it does not come in contact with dirt.

A bacteriologist named Soxhlet, in 1882, finding that a certain degree of heat would kill germs, proposed a simple method of heating milk, and it was believed for a time that the problem was solved. During the next twenty years, however, with sterilization widely practiced, the death-rate among infants declined very little.

Then it was discovered that heating the milk, while it killed the germs, caused changes in the proteids, salts, fats and other constituents, and that the products of such changes were often dangerous. It was also found that the constituents of cow's milk differ vastly from those of mother's milk, and that some of them in their natural state are poisonous to human infants. The result was an effort to change these constituents in such a way that they would more closely resemble the corresponding constituents of mother's milk. This effort is still in progress, and its visible fruit is the large number of "modified" milks now offered. Some of these are excellent, and, if properly administered, almost all of them do more good than harm, but we are still far from a modified cow's milk which exactly duplicates mother's milk. This is proved by the fact that, despite the progress made, the death-rate among bottle-fed babies exceeds by far that among babies fed at the breast. Both have declined enormously in the past twenty years, but that decline is due not so much to improvements in food as to improvements in the prevention and treatment of contaminated milk and the diseases it produces.

A gigantic hoard of ancient fallacies and superstitions clusters about the nursing mother. There are a thousand signs and portents which command immediate weaning, and I suspect that, in the case of many of them, the wish is father to the too-ready belief. All sorts of slight indispositions are seized upon as excuses for condemning the baby to the bottle—a trifling cold, a temporary reduction in the quantity of milk, a day or two of poor appetite, a headache, even a toothache. "That tired feeling," accompanied by irregularities in the milk-supply, is often the effect of a night at the theatre, a game of bridge or an attempt at heavy housework. The nursing mother must take good care of herself, she must keep early hours, get plenty of sleep and food, and avoid all emotional excitement, but she is by no means an invalid, and those slight aches and illnesses which afflict all of us incessantly do not afford her a sound reason for neglecting her sacred obligation to her child and to the human race. I have succeeded in bringing milk back into women's breasts who had not nursed the child for three months.

It is commonly believed that if the nursing mother, for some minor indisposition, takes a drug of any sort, it will appear in the milk and injure the child. In the main, this is not true. Very few drugs do this, and it is easy for the mother to avoid those. Among them are codeine, salicylic acid and mercury. The last is not frequently prescribed, but the first is contained in many patent "headache cures," and the second is often used to preserve canned foods. It is easy enough to avoid "headache powders" and it is easy, too, to avoid canned foods. Even in case the latter are eaten, it is possible to avoid those which contain salicylic acid, for the presence of this drug, thanks to the new pure food law, must now be announced upon the label.

The nursing mother would better eschew all stimulants, but if she has been in the habit of drinking, say, a glass of beer a day, there is no reason why she should stop it during the nursing period. I am no apologist for alcohol, but it is an undoubted fact that those who are habituated to it, in small quantities, suffer discomfort on abandoning its use, and this discomfort may imperil the milk-supply far more than the alcohol itself.

The old notion that a bottle of beer, ale or porter a day benefits mother and child by "strengthening" the former and increasing the supply of milk is an utterly nonsensical superstition. Far from being strengthening, beer is the very reverse, and ale and porter, having more alcohol in them, are even worse. Therefore, it is dangerous for any woman to begin their use during the nursing period, but, all the same, it is inadvisable for a women who has grown accustomed to them to abandon them suddenly.

The same thing may be said of tea and coffee. The woman who has looked forward daily to her afternoon cup of tea cannot forswear it without discomfort, and this emotional storm may easily interfere with the milk-supply. Such a woman needs her cup of tea as much as a smoker needs his afterdinner cigar. As every one knows, the smoker who tries to stop smoking suddenly often suffers agonies which bring him to the verge of an actual nervous breakdown.

But in all such matters it is wise to exercise great moderation. Beer, tea and coffee must ever be regarded not as necessary foods, but as necessary evils. The woman who employs stimulants to enable her to perform the double task of nursing a baby and doing heavy housework is very short-sighted, to say the least. Within a short time the penalty will have to be paid—and the poor baby, unluckily, will have to pay most of it.

Best of all stimulants and auxiliaries for nursing mothers is clean, fresh cow's milk. An adult woman, in most cases, is able to digest it without discomfort. Its nourishing constituents will give her healthy blood and general well-being, and these boons she will pass on to her child. This is the best of all methods of modifying cow's milk for infant consumption, and the wizards of the laboratory will never produce anything to equal it.

Commentary

Chapter 6: The Bottle-Fed Baby and **Chapter 7: A Chapter on Milk**

The Battle of the Bottle: A Brief History of Infant Nutrition

The subject of infant feeding seems somewhat hackneyed in these sophisticated days and perhaps for that reason more than any other needs occasional appraisal and reorientation.[1]

So wrote Grover Francis Powers, M.D., Professor of Pediatrics at the Yale Medical School, in the lead article of the *Journal of the American Medical Association's* September 7, 1935 issue. And the reappraisal is still going on.

The interest among physicians in the artificial feeding of infants was largely responsible for the emergence of pediatrics from general internal medicine as a separate medical specialty. The intricate modified cow-milk formulas prescribed for infants were so complex that general practitioners sometimes had to consult a specialist in infant nutrition who was facile with the manipulations of fats, protein, and carbohydrates. To make these matters of feeding even more confusing, each prominent professor of pediatrics at every leading medical center in the United States, Germany, and France seemed to have his own formula for bottlefeeding that was "superior" to all others.

"The Bottle-Fed Baby" and "A Chapter on Milk" reiterate Mencken and Hirshberg's staunch conviction that human breast milk is superior to formula. As Mencken states, "the wizards of the laboratory will never produce anything equal to it." On the other hand, the chapters do acknowledge situations in which breastfeeding is unwise or impractical and offer counsel on proper bottlefeeding and formula preparation. The movement in pediatrics to create acceptable artificial formulas for infants was instrumental in the decline of infant mortality from the 1900s to the present. It resulted in the easy accessibility of processed, pasteurized, and germ-free infant milk products that set hygienic standards for the entire dairy industry. Understanding the rather vigorous debate of breastfeeding versus bottlefeeding beyond the axioms "breast is best" and "cow's milk is for calves," requires a glimpse at the development of artificial feeding for infants.

Until approximately the 18th century, the most widely used and reliable source of infant nutrition was human breast milk. Soranus of Ephesus, a Greek physician of the second century, is credited for innovating the "fingernail technique," a method for analyzing the freshness of breast milk that was used for over 15 centuries:

> That Mylke is goode that is whyte and sweete; and when ye droppe it on your nail and do not move your finger, neyther fleteth abrod at every stirring nor will hange faste upon your nayle, when ye turne it downward, but that whyche is betwene both is safe.[2]

Although breastfeeding was the principal means of infant nutrition, especially among the poorer classes, until the 1900s, breastfeeding and childrearing were hardly considered desirable duties by parents from Antiquity to the Middle Ages. Children were poorly understood as being "tiny adults" and were neither highly regarded nor valued. As late as the 13th century, for example, infanticide and abandonment were accepted and common means of getting rid of unwanted babies. These abusive practices were gradually refined in Europe during the Enlightment (the 18th century), when parents routinely sent the infant soon after delivery to a wet nurse for its nutrition. Upon weaning, many sent their children to monasteries and convents or, if the parents were poor, to foster families as slaves or indentured servants. In 18th century France, for example, uneasy parents, nervous about or afraid of caring for a frail infant, were all too eager to obtain the services of a wet nurse. The wet-nursing industry boomed in France and soon spread to Great Britain during the 1700s and early 1800s, despite protests from physicians who warned about the higher incidence of contagious illnesses among infants with wet nurses. If a family could not afford a wet nurse and the mother could not breastfeed, the infant was often fed pap and panada, mixtures of flour, milk, water and alcohol or an opiate, through special devices called pap-spoons.

Even in the early 1800s, however, physicians had begun to accumulate evidence that breastfed babies grew healthier and quicker than those fed exclusively pap or cow's milk. Babies fed only pap were described as "atrophic," pale, and sickly. The infants with wet-nurses, despite their slightly higher incidence of infections than infants who were nursed by their mothers, fared better than "artificially-fed" infants. In fact, the initial failures of bottlefeeding (i.e., with pap or unmodified cow's milk) led it to be all but abandoned during the 19th century, as recalled by pediatrician-historian Thomas E. Cone:

> Throughout almost the entire 19th century, pessimistic opinions about the fate of bottle fed infants prevailed, and many 19th century reports indicated that among infants who were not breastfed, as many as 80 to 90% died. In the New York Foundling Asylum, bottle fed infants were kept to themselves in a room known as the ward of the dying babies, and in the foundling home located on Randall's Island in New York City, only one bottle fed infant admitted to the hospital in the period of a year and a half during the 1880's had reached the age of one year.[3]

Before bottlefeeding was to be accepted as the major means of infant feeding of the 20th century, there were two large scientific problems that needed to be resolved. The most pressing problem was eliminating the high bacteria counts routinely found in raw, unrefrigerated milk, a food that could kill its young consumers if not handled scrupulously well. Although Mencken slightly misquotes a line from John Milton's poem *Il Penseroso*, he makes an excellent point on the ability of improperly handled milk to cause disease:

> When a cow is milked the milk takes up floating germs from the air, through which it passes in its descent to the can, just as the raindrops of a Summer shower take upon "the gay motes that dance along a sunbeam."[4] These germs, finding milk a fertile soil, begin to multiply at once and with enormous rapidity.... If the can is unclean, or has been washed with contaminated water, if the milkman had dirty hands, or if the cow itself is infected with tuberculosis or any other infectious disease, other and more virulent germs reinforce those of the air, and before long the innocent-appearing can of milk is swarming with organisms.

"Tainted milk" was a common problem prior to the advent of refrigeration in the 1920s. Each June or July brought epidemics of "infantile summer diarrhea" (gastroenteritis) and made diarrhea and dehydration leading causes of infant mortality. As the 19th century closed, however, many advances in milk sterilization had occurred, elevating bottlefeeding from folly to the feasible. In 1864 Louis Pasteur developed the process that bears his name in order to save France's ailing wine industry from the huge losses incurred by wine spoilage. Pasteurization was eventually applied to milk and is still the best way to eliminate pathogenic (disease-producing) bacteria without altering taste by heating the milk to a constant temperature of 60°C in a special apparatus. Pasteurization of milk did not become popular until the first decade of the 20th century because it was expensive, difficult, and required a hard-to-obtain apparatus. Mencken and Hirshberg note the more popular and simple method of sterilizing milk described by Franz von Soxhlet in 1886.[5] Soxhlet's sterilization process called for boiling milk at 100°C for 1½ hours and, like pasteurization, was shown to rid milk of typhoid, dysentery, tuberculosis, and streptococci. The creation of large, hygienic milk laboratories in New York, Boston, and other major cities beginning in 1889 led to the widespread use of pasteurization for milk sterilization in the United States. The milk laboratories would both sterilize the milk and modify it according to physician's prescription.[6]

With the problem of milk sterilization solved, food companies were anxious to bring infant formulas, the newly developed condensed milk, and "pocket wet nurses" to the market. Interestingly, the milk industry was not the only food industry that cleaned up its system of operations during this period. Having become aware of the possibility of ingesting tainted, spoiled, or improperly handled food, the public demanded laws to protect their interests. Soon the food chain came under protection by federal legislation, specifically the Pure Food and Drug Act of 1906 and the Meat Inspection Act of 1907. The subsequent discoveries of vitamins A, B, C, and D and the addition of iodine to table salt (for prevention of endemic goiter) all helped give rise to the science of nutrition and a public convinced of the importance of a balanced diet "fortified" with vitamins, minerals, and trace elements. By 1925 "nutritious" prepared foods, including artificial infant formula, had mass-market appeal. Nutrition was not only a burgeoning scientific field, but it was also perceived by the public as a means of ridding society of its diseases.

The second problem of artificial feeding that required investigation had to do with the proteid (protein), fat, and carbohydrate content in milk. Recall that in the early 1800s, infants fed exclusively cow milk developed rather poorly in comparison to their breastfed counterparts. One explanation for the poor results with cow milk was offered by J. Franz Simon in 1838 and Philip Biedert in 1869. These German pediatricians believed that cow milk needed to be modified so that it contained the same percentages of fat, proteins, and carbohydrates as human breast milk. Mencken muses that cow milk protein coagulates like a fried egg compared to the "fine flakes [of a mother's milk protein] which remain separate and are easily attacked by the secretion of the baby's stomach." This theory occupied the minds of many physicians, including L. Emmett Holt, who noted in 1907:

> The first dense coagulum which forms with cow's milk is greatly lessened by diluting the milk, but does not disappear altogether even when the total proteins are made the same as in mother's milk.[7]

In 1903 Dr. Thomas Morgan Rotch, who held Harvard's newly created chair of Pediatrics, introduced the German or percentage method of infant feeding to American physicians. Rotch, too, held that the major protein of cow milk, casein, was far more difficult for an infant to digest than the major protein of human milk, lactalbumin. Rotch proposed diluting the milk formula with water; the amount of dilution was, theoretically, based on the infant's age and tolerance. Many American pediatricians followed Rotch's theories on artificial feeding and began experimenting with the percentage method in order to prescribe the ideal artificial formula for each infant.

As pediatricians and food chemists became more facile in their analysis of milk constituents and confident in their abilities to overcome the differences between cow-milk formulas and human milk, variations on the theme of the percentage method began to emerge. Each variation, often far more subtle than what the heated arguments surrounding them indicated, was heralded in the medical literature as "*the* artificial formula" to use. Czerny, Finkelstein, Biedert, Meigs, Rotch, Holt, Cowie, and a number of other prominent pediatricians each held steadfastly to his own formula. Dr. Grover Powers observed the "strict dogmatic attitude" of pediatricians applying the science of nutrition to infant feeding. Powers characterized this attitude as "the itch for perfection in dietary regimen—as a direct result of the propaganda for weighing and measuring—in short, for standardization."[8]

Standard infant formulas began to be mass produced in sophisticated, sterile milk laboratories in the 1920s. The product's introduction to the market coincided with the wide national interest in nutrition and clean foodstuffs described above. Taken in the context of the times, the nutrition movement, the woman's suffrage movement, the loosening of a moral and social structure in which men clearly dominated women, and the amount of freedom offered by a bottle in contrast to the confinement of breastfeeding all contributed to making bottlefeeding an old idea whose time had come.

Today, the pediatrician can offer a number of carefully developed and properly prepared infant formulas that simulate human milk. Products with names such as Similac and SMA (cow milk–based formulas) or Prosobee and Isomil (soy milk–based formulas) can be conveniently purchased in the supermarket or drug store and are easily prepared in the home. More complex formulas can be prescribed that are specially prepared for infants with digestive or metabolic disorders. Artificial formulas are clean, standardized, and convenient alternatives to breastfeeding and are firmly entrenched as the most popular method of feeding infants in the United States today.

Drinking and Breastfeeding Redux

In contrast to the strict warnings in the article "Mother and Baby" against breastfeeding mothers imbibing alcohol or caffeine, a more temperate Mencken closes "A Chapter on Milk" by offering mild reassurance for the mother who drinks perhaps one glass of beer a day: "I am no apologist for alcohol, but it is an undisputed fact that those who are habituated to it ... suffer discomfort on abandoning its use, and this discomfort may imperil the milk supply far more than the alcohol itself...."

Although Mencken was not an alcoholic, he enjoyed drinking in the spirit of comraderie and for relaxation. A member of several "drinking clubs" throughout his adult life and an aficionado of good beer, Mencken often quipped: "I've made it a rule never to drink by daylight and never to refuse a drink after dark." Hirshberg also had a passion for good German beer. The physician was noted in Baltimore for, among other things, his annual Thanksgiving parties featuring guests such as Mencken and Mr. and Mrs. Theodore Dreiser and "beer and Meyerbeer."[9]

Consuming alcohol is never recommended during pregnancy or nursing. The risk of adverse effects on the developing fetus is high when an expectant mother drinks alcohol in significant quantities. Alcohol has an association with specific defects collectively called the fetal-alcohol syndrome, which includes mental retardation, growth retardation, and a characteristic facial appearance. In the case of the nursing mother who is a chronic drinker or alcoholic, Mencken's assessment is correct that abrupt abstention may be more deleterious than continued moderate consumption owing to the debilitating effects of withdrawal. Such a mother would most likely be urged to bottlefeed and encouraged to obtain counselling for her alcohol problem.

Mencken and Hirshberg sympathize with nursing mothers about the problem of caffeine addiction: "Such a woman needs her cup of tea as a smoker needs his after dinner cigar." Some scientific data link hyperactive behavior in breastfed babies to the amount of caffeine consumed by breastfeeding mothers. Thus, most pediatricians recommend elimination of caffeine-containing beverages (e.g., coffee, tea, soft drinks, etc.) from the nursing mother's diet. The chapter closes with an excellent summation of the effect of drugs, medications, and alcohol on the nursing mother:

> But in all such matters it is wise to exercise great moderation. Beer, tea, and coffee must ever be regarded not as necessary foods but as necessary evils.

To this we would add a phrase so frequently heard it has become a cliche: "Consult your physician."

QUESTIONS FOR THE MOTHER ABOUT CHAPTER 6

1. Why is it that so many more bottle-fed babies get sick and die than breast-fed babies?

1910 Babies often have diarrhea and vomit because the milk is not clean—has not been kept cold—has been kept too long—is not properly prepared or the nursing bottles and nipples are dirty.

Current Today in developed countries there is no demonstrated difference in mortality rates between bottlefed and breastfed babies, although a difference remains with respect to the incidence of otitis media, upper respiratory tract infections, and certain forms of infectious diarrhea between breastfed and bottlefed infants. Breast milk appears to confer protection for a variety of reasons, some of which are poorly understood even today. Human milk is rich in antibodies and also contains leukocytes, lymphocytes and all the components of the complement system, and lysozyme. In additon human milk apparently has substances, presumably polysaccharides, that interfere with bacterial attachment to epithelial surfaces that line the respiratory, gastrointestinal, and urinary tracts of the infant. Breast milk is still regarded by many as having mysterious properties that promote good health.

2. How can a mother avoid the danger that comes to babies through cow's milk?

1910 She could consult a doctor that knows about babies, and find out if she can not nurse the child. If not, she should get from her doctor a prescription for preparing the milk to suit her baby's stomach. She should weigh her baby on the same scales once a week, and if she finds the child losing weight or not gaining for several weeks, she should consult her doctor again and ask that the formula be changed.

Current The mother can avoid any problems that could be caused by the feeding of whole cow milk by following the recommendation of the Committee on Nutrition of the American Academy of Pediatrics, which advises against the feeding of whole cow milk to any infant during the first 6 months of life.

3. What is the best and easiest way to prepare the milk?

1910 The milk should be prepared every morning for the day's supply. It should be put into the feeding bottles and corked with aseptic cotton and put on the ice. Each bottle should be warmed by putting the bottle in hot water just before giving it to the baby. The bottles should be boiled just before filling with the day's milk. Throw away what the baby leaves. Never give the leftover milk to it for another feeding. As soon as the bottle used by the baby is empty, it should be thoroughly washed with cold water—then cleansed with borax and hot water (one teaspoonful of borax to a pint of water). The nipple should be thoroughly washed after each nursing with hot water and when not in use should soak in boric water in a covered glass. The nipple must be rinsed in boiling water just before the baby uses it. Bottles and nipples should be boiled once a day.

Current The principles described in 1910 are still applicable today, although scrupulous sterilization of the formula is not required in most communities because of the improved nature of the water supply. The feeding of prepared proprietary formulas to the non-breastfed infant totally eliminates the need for the precautions described in 1910.

4. Why need such extreme care be taken to sterilize bottles and nipples before giving them to the baby?

1910 Because milk is one of the best "culture" mediums. Germs develop in milk with incredible rapidity. Therefore you may often be giving poison to your baby when you think you are giving it clean, nourishing milk.

Current Milk is still regarded as an excellent culture medium, particularly when the milk is not kept refrigerated or is mixed with a contaminated water supply.

5. What should a mother do if her baby has diarrhea?

1910 Diarrhea comes from too much food—too frequent feeding—too little water—too little sleep—too much handling—too little air, and *from milk that is dirty or has not been kept on ice.*

Current In the United States today, diarrhea most commonly results from a viral infection of the gastrointestinal tract or secondary to an infection in other parts of the body. If an infant has diarrhea while being breastfed, breastfeeding should be continued. If a non-breastfed infant develops diarrhea, consideration should be given to a temporary cessation of formula feeding and substitution of an electrolyte and glucose containing fluid. If diarrhea continues, a physician should be consulted.

6. Why does a child vomit and have diarrhea?

1910 Because some food that it cannot digest, some sour or dirty milk has been taken into its stomach, and it vomits and has diarrhea because it is trying to get rid of the food that is making it sick.

Current Both vomiting and diarrhea are usually caused by an infection but may be due to excessive feeding or poor techniques of bottlefeeding that result in the infant's swallowing too much air. It is unusual today in the United States for infants to develop vomiting or diarrhea because of intolerance to the proprietary formula.

7. Why does diarrhea come to babies in summer?

1910 Because in summer milk gets warm, and germs and poisons multiply.

Current Because certain viral infections of the gastrointestinal tract are more common in the summer months, although the most commonly recognized viral cause of diarrhea, rotavirus, is actually prevalent in winter months in this country.

8. Why do more bottle-fed than breast-fed babies have diarrhea?

1910 Because cow's milk is less likely to be pure and suited to the baby's stomach than mother's milk.

Current Because breast milk contains substances that reduce the risk of an infant developing an infection of the gastrointestinal tract that results in diarrhea.

9. How can a mother prevent diarrhea?

1910 By taking a baby to her doctor to be sure its food is right before hot weather sets in—by keeping it out in the fresh air, bathing it daily and sponging it with cool water on hot days—by keeping it quiet and letting it have plenty of sleep. Thus its body will be able to resist disease.

Current By breastfeeding her baby during the first 6 months of life and by reducing contact with other infants who are experiencing an infectious diarrhea.

QUESTIONS FOR THE MOTHER ABOUT CHAPTER 7

1. Why is mother's milk better for young babies than cow's milk?

1910 Nature has put all the elements necessary to nourish and develop the baby in the milk of a healthy mother.

Current Human milk is a complete food for infants if the mother is well-nourished. The baby who is fed cow milk must receive supplements of vitamins A and C and the milk must be fortified with vitamin D in order to compensate for the deficiencies in cow milk. The iron in human milk is readily absorbed and will meet the iron needs of the exclusively breastfed infant for the first 6 to 9 months of life, whereas the infant receiving cow milk must be provided with an iron supplement in order to prevent iron deficiency anemia. Human milk contains immunologic substances that reduce the risk of infection in the breastfed baby, whereas cow's milk is devoid of such protective material, at least for humans.

2. Why must cow's milk be modified for babies?

1910 It must be made as nearly as possible like mother's milk.

Current Because it contains too much protein for the young infant, too much salt, too much phosphorus, and has a fat that is poorly absorbed by babies. The protein of cow milk tends to curdle or form a coagulum in the infant's stomach, which can result in intestinal obstruction. Heating, acidifying, or diluting the whole cow milk serves to reduce its curd-forming capability. Unmodified cow milk also induces subtle gastrointestinal bleeding in many infants during the first year of life. Heat treatment of the milk alters the protein and reduces its capability to induce bleeding.

3. Why will not the same formula do for all babies?

1910 Each mother's milk is different, suited to the particular needs of her baby. No two babies' stomachs are exactly alike. Therefore, the doctor makes an analysis of a mother's milk to find out just how to prepare the artificial food for her baby. Often when he finds out what is lacking in the mother's milk, he can, by special diet in the matter, rectify her milk or supplement the absent ingredients by giving the baby one bottle-feeding a day.

Current The proprietary formulas of today, unlike the formulas concocted by physicians in 1910, can be fed to almost all infants. Special formulas have been developed for small premature infants, but term infants can be given one of the standard formulas. Most commercial formulas are very similar in basic composition.

4. Why must the baby's formula be frequently changed?

1910 Because the baby's stomach develops and requires different ingredients to continue the development. Nature varies mother's milk to suit the baby's developing stomach.

Current Except for the growing premature infant, the formula fed to the term infant does not have to be changed frequently—in fact, it does not have to be changed at all during the first year of life.

5. Why is pasteurized milk often recommended for babies?

1910 Because many bacteriologists believe that pasteurization kills the germs in milk that make babies sick.

Current Because pasteurization destroys bacteria that may produce diarrhea and other forms of infection. The pasteurization process also kills the tubercle bacillus. In 1910, babies fed unpasteurized milk from infected cows often ended up with tuberculosis.

6. What is pasteurization?

1910 It is raising milk to a temperature of from 140 to 167 degrees Fahrenheit and keeping it at that temperature for from 20 to 30 minutes.

Current The process is still the same.

7. How is it that pasteurization does not kill the germs in milk that nourish the "favorable" germs?

1910 There is no reason to believe that it does not. Does this not work an injury to the baby? Many physicians believe that it does. Many also believe that this is a lesser evil than impure milk.

Current Pasteurization, when performed properly, kills all bacteria.

8. Is there no way of procuring raw milk that is safe?

1910 Yes, milk that is carefully and intelligently produced is safe for the baby to take raw if properly modified.

Current No.

9. How may a mother know if raw milk is safe?

1910 She may have her board of health make frequent bacteriological tests of the milk coming from the dairy. She may visit the farm and inspect the methods of producing milk.

Current There is no way to ensure the absolute safety of unpasteurized milk in sufficient time to have fresh milk to drink.

10. What are some of the things up-to-date dairymen do to protect milk?

1910 They keep the cows in a well-aired, clean smelling cow-barn. They feed cows clean, good food. They have their men wear clean white milking suits. They have the cows' bellies and udders washed in disinfectant and the men wash their hands in disinfectant before milking. They have all bottles thoroughly sterilized. They have milk immediately cooled and kept at 50 degrees Fahrenheit until it reaches the consumer.

Current The same safety procedures are followed today but dairymen depend on pasteurization to produce a safe product.

11. Does not this increase the cost of producing milk?

1910 Yes, every mother should be willing to pay extra to have the best milk. Milk that is fit for babies cannot be produced under 8 cents a quart. *Beware of 5 cent milk. Beware of "loose" milk.*

Current Good sanitary procedures do increase the cost of milk. The cost of milk, however, is kept artificially high because the government maintains the price by buying milk when the price begins to fall.

12. Is not 10 or 15 cents a quart for milk for your baby cheaper than letting it get sick and perhaps die?

1910 Yes, you pay it not only for your baby but for all babies. Every time a mother buys cheap milk she makes it harder for dairymen to produce good, clean milk. The realization of this fact by mothers will do more than any other thing to secure a universally safe milk supply.

Current Milk costs far more today. The price of a proprietary infant formula with its added vitamins and minerals is almost the same as the price of whole milk, and it should be fed to infants who are not being breastfed for the first year of life. Saving money by feeding an infant cow milk is a false economy and should be avoided.

13. Must milk be always kept at 50 degrees Fahrenheit?

1910 Yes. It is better to get a small supply twice a day if you have no ice. A small piece of ice in water will keep bottles cold all day and sometimes longer. If you cannot get ice, wrap a cloth wrung out in cold water around the milk bottle. Always keep milk covered. If you know that the milk has been warmer than 50°F. for long, then boil it before using it.

Current Cow milk should be kept refrigerated at 40 degrees Fahrenheit. Proprietary formulas should also be kept refrigerated once the bottle has been opened or the powdered formula prepared.

REFERENCES

1. Powers GF. Infant nutrition: Historical background and modern practice. *Journal of the American Medical Association* 105:753–761, 1935.
2. Still GF. *The History of Paediatrics*. London: Oxford University Press, 1931, pp. 29–30.
3. Cone TE. History of infant feeding (with special emphasis on the United States). *In* Rudolph AM (ed.). *Pediatrics* (17th ed.) New York: Appleton-Century-Crofts, 1982, pp. 167–169.
4. Milton wrote the line: "the gay motes that people a sunbeam." *Il Penseroso,* line 8. *In* Milton J. *Complete Poems and Major Prose*. Indianapolis: Odyssey Press, 1978, pp. 72–76.
5. Mencken and Hirshberg incorrectly cite von Soxhlet's discovery as occurring in 1882 but it actually was reported in 1886. See Soxhlet F. *Munchen Med. Wochenschr.* 33:253–276, 1886.
6. In 1889, Dr. Henry Koplik set up the first gouttes de lait or "milk depot" in the U.S. at the Good Samaritan Dispensary in New York City. Here, Koplik "bought the best bottled milk, sterilized it in separate portions, and thus did the very best for my patients" (see Koplik H. The history of milk depots or gouttes de lait in the U.S. *Journal of the American Medical Association* 63:1574–1575, 1914). By 1891, the Walker-Gordon Milk Laboratory in Boston was offering "pure, clean milk" to the public.
7. Holt LE. *Diseases of Infancy and Childhood* (3rd ed.). New York: D. Appleton and Co., 1907, p. 183.
8. Powers GF. *Journal of the American Medical Association* 105:753–761, 1935.
9. Mencken to Dreiser, 15 November 1909, The Theodore Dreiser Collection, Special Collections, Van Pelt Library, University of Pennsylvania, Philadelphia, Pa.

8
The Food for Growing Children

Toward the end of the first year a human infant begins to be the most interesting thing in the world. Heretofore it has lived a life of colorless, unconscious, vegetative growth; and though its mother, perhaps, has discerned a meaning and a portent in its every sign, its actions, in sober truth, have been chiefly *re*-actions, and, as such, have sadly lacked motive and coherence. But now its intelligence is dawning and the mysterious something that we call personality is unfolding. It begins to differ from other babies of its age in a thousand surprising and delightful ways; it acquires habits, appetites, little vanities, likes and dislikes, and what may be called a customary attitude of mind. And these things appear, one after the other, with truly dazzling rapidity. Every week sees noticeable progress. Every day has its perceptible change.

Mind and body join in the metamorphosis. Muscular and organic activity increases, and a multitude of ideas—nebulous, maybe, but still vastly engaging—begin to throng the child's brain. It begins to take note of the world about it; to recognize differences; to observe cause and effect; to put fact and fact together. And with all this awakening from within there comes a need of changes without.

As every woman knows, the time for weaning commonly brings perils for the infant. That this is the rule is shown by the fact that popular lore has given it the dignity of an immutable law of nature. As a matter of fact, there is no reason whatever why weaning should bring serious consequences to either mother or child, for it is as thoroughly normal an incident of life as birth or teething. In practically all cases the disasters of this period are due to an inaccurate reading of the baby's needs.

Many mothers believe that a prolongation of nursing is beneficial to the child, but this is not true. The baby fed upon milk exclusively beyond the normal time is usually a weak and anemic child, whose external appearance gives evidence of the retarded development of its organs of assimilation.

Until it is well on toward its second birthday, the principal food of every child should be milk, but this milk needs reinforcement. Let one meal be of modified cow's milk alone, and the next of milk and toast, with milk next and then a bit of mashed potato, and so on.

In this connection, and before proceeding to a consideration of the diet later on, it may be well to point out that the dietary needs of every child are determined more by its weight than by its age. An average baby, weighing about eight pounds at birth, should weigh about seventeen pounds at the age of nine months, when it is ready to be weaned. If it weighs less than this, it is well to seek medical advice before making changes in its food.

The same factor determines the amount of food required by the child each day. A normal baby of twelve months, weighing twenty-one pounds, will need five feedings of modified cow's milk, of eight ounces each and at intervals of four hours, in addition to the alternate meals of toast, rice, and so on. But if the child weighs but sixteen or seventeen pounds, six or seven ounces of milk will be sufficient. By the same token, if it weighs more than twenty-one pounds, it may well take a bit more than eight ounces.

Once the milk of early infancy has been reinforced by the starchy foods, and the child has passed the Rubicon in safety, it is in order to reduce the former, by slow stages, to second place. As soon as possible teach the child to drink from a cup and give it its daily milk in that way. Reduce its allowance of milk to four eight-ounce rations a day, and at the same time add a meal of beef-juice or mutton-broth with a soft-boiled or poached egg. By the time the child is a year and a half old, broiled and scraped steak may be substituted for the broths.

To prepare this sear a round steak, on the outside only, over a brisk fire and scrape it into a fine pulp with a knife. Take about two tablespoonfuls of this and mix it thoroughly with an equal amount of stale bread-crumbs. Then let the baby eat it with a spoon.

Toward the end of the second year it is time to abandon the

schedule of meals I have given in a previous chapter, and to progress, by degrees, toward three a day. Begin by omitting the meal of milk taken just before bedtime and gradually increase the importance of the midday dinner. By this time the baby will begin diet by the addition of roasts and chops, poultry and fish, but it is well to serve all of these things finely chopped until the fifth or sixth year, since all children, even when their teeth are equal to the task of masticating meats, are likely to bolt them without proper chewing. The daily allowance should be not more than a few ounces, and it should be reduced on the first indication of digestive disturbance.

Needless to say, all forms of pork are dangerous, and no child should taste the flesh of the swine until its eighth or ninth year, at least. In particular, such things as bacon, ham, shoulder and sausage should be avoided, and the same may be said of all parts of beef, mutton and poultry, save the finest cuts. A child's stomach is ill fitted for the digestion of giblet-stew, liver and bacon, sour beef, calves-head, bologna sausage, pigs' feet and other such delicatessen. Similarly, it can ill cope with fried chops or fried fish. The best meats for it are beef and mutton, boiled, broiled or roasted, and the best fish are larger ones, which may be boiled or baked. Under poultry I include chicken (broiled or baked, but never fried), roast turkey and roast barn-yard duck.

Many mothers are under the impression that all vegetables, without exception, have excellent dietetic and medicinal virtues, but this is not true, even in the case of adults. With children it is well to avoid all save those which may be boiled for several hours, and to make a further extension of the ban to cabbage sprouts and corn. The vegetables which enter into a meat stew, such as potatoes, carrots, turnips and onions, all well boiled, are nourishing and harmless, and the same is true of spinach. But is must be remembered here that "well boiled" should be taken literally. It is not sufficient to boil carrots until they are tender. Instead, they must be cooked to pieces.

Of all the fruits which may enter into the midday dinner the apple, peeled, baked and seeded, is by far the best. After it come its near relatives, the pear and peach. It is well to bake or stew all three before giving them to children, at least until the age of six or seven years, but the juice of the peach, without the pulp, is harmless. In the same way, the juices of tamarinds, grapefruit and pineapples may be fed to children, even as early as the third year, with safety and benefit, whereas all of these fruits, eaten in the ordinary way, are exceedingly dangerous. It is true enough that many children eat them, but it is also true enough that many children die of cholera infantum and diarrhea.

They harbor germs, their woody pulp is indigestible, and some have numerous seeds. Cherries and the smaller berries are undesirable also, and bananas, while seedless and germless, overburden the stomach.

The third meal of a child's day, taken in early evening, should be much like its breakfast, save in the absence of the morning egg. Milk and toast or milk and a cereal should constitute its mainstay, with a cupful of milk added. At these two milk-meals no meat, vegetable or fruit should be served. Until its eighth or ninth year a child should never eat meat more than once a day, and no fruits should be served when milk is on the table.

As soon as the three-meal-a-day schedule has been established the child should be refused all solid food between meals, but it is a good custom throughout childhood—and necessary until the seventh year—to give a generous cupful of milk in the middle of the morning and another in the middle of the afternoon. If the child is hungry, let it drink two cupfuls, and, on the other hand, do not press it to drink if it is not so disposed, as the appetites of children vary as much as those of adults.

In conclusion, remember this: that until it is fourteen a child is not capable of dealing with the miscellaneous mass which makes up the civilized bill of fare. If it must eat at the family table, see that its share of the dishes is rigorously limited. Discourage the use of coffee, chocolate and tea, and give it little, if any, pork in any form. Hot rolls, waffles, pancakes and other things of that sort, are always dangerous.

In the matter of candies and other sweets exercise a stern censorship. If it were possible, it would be well for the children of the land to grow up in ignorance of these delights. Nevertheless, every mother may do much to discourage the ancient custom of making candy a reward for diligence and good order. A child however needs some sugar and should have a little on its food.

Commentary

Chapter 8: The Food for Growing Children

If the feeding practices expounded by Mencken and Hirshberg were followed today, the infant would still grow up healthy. However, their recommendations are unnecessarily rigid and would not lead to mealtime enjoyment or to the development of good lifetime nutritional habits. The diets recommended were prepared by Dr. Charles Chapin in 1909. They are essentially identical to the diets recommended by L.

Emmett Holt in *The Care and Feeding of Children*. Strict control of the infant, including what the baby ate, was customary in those days. It is instructive to compare Mencken's recommendations for the feeding of infants and toddlers with current recommendations from the Committee on Nutrition of the American Academy of Pediatrics.

1. The newborn infant The authors of *What You Ought to Know About Your Baby* and the American Academy of Pediatrics both assert that human milk is the optimal food for the infant. The American Academy of Pediatrics maintains that breast milk or an iron-fortified formula, a product not available in 1910, can provide all the nutritional needs for most full-term infants until the infant's weight reaches 6 to 7 kg (13 to 15 pounds). Current recommendations call for the avoidance of whole cow milk for the first 6 months of life, and many believe that unmodified whole cow milk should not be given to infants until after the first year of life. Solid foods need not be introduced until the infant reaches 5 to 7 months of age. The early introduction of solid foods is believed to put the infant at risk for the development of gastrointestinal allergy and possible obesity.

2. Introducing solid foods: the 6-month-old infant Like Mencken and Hirshberg, the Academy holds that there is no known nutritional basis for starting solid foods before 3 months of age. The Committee on Nutrition states that, "By waiting until this time, it is usually possible to avoid or minimize feeding problems caused by lack of neuromuscular readiness for solid feeding, chronic overeating, parental anxiety, and food intolerance and allergy."[1]

The goal of nutrition, particularly in infancy, is to support optimal growth, prevent deficiencies, prevent later disease as a consequence of early feeding practices, and establish good feeding habits by preventing the development of food preferences for sugar, salt and fatty foods. The Committee on Nutrition has developed the following guidelines for the introduction of solid foods:

1. Attempt to make every mealtime a pleasant social experience.
2. Start foods other than formula when the infant weighs 6 to 7 kg (note that Mencken also used weight rather than age as a guide to the introduction of solid food).
3. Start with small serving sizes of 1 to 2 teaspoonfuls, increasing gradually to 3 to 4 tablespoonfuls per feeding.
4. Introduce single-ingredient foods one at a time and continue for 5 days before introducing another food. This recommendation is designed to recognize early food intolerance.

It is common practice, among pediatricians, to introduce rice cereal first, then fruits, then vegetables, and finally meats. Juices are also introduced one at a time. This order of food introduction, like Mencken's, is based on common sense rather than on scientific data.

3. Feeding the toddler The Nutrition Committee, like Mencken and Hirshberg, recommend that a diet plan be established for the older infant which includes the "basic four food groups" for balance and diversity. The "basic four" food groups are milk, meat, bread and cereals, and fruits and vegetables. The intake of whole milk should be limited to 720 ml, or three 8-ounce glasses, per day.

Most pediatricians would endorse Mencken's advice that the child be taught to drink from the cup by the end of the first year of life and that egg whites should be avoided during the first year of life because of their allergic potential. However, it is no longer true that "all forms of pork are dangerous." Similarly, no pediatrician would recommend boiling vegetables for several hours before feeding them to a child. It is now recognized that vegetables that are "cooked to pieces" lose most of their nutritional value.

The infant at 2 years of age is believed to be capable of eating most, if not all, foods eaten by the older family members, although in smaller portions. The foods forbidden by Mencken and Hirshberg are not prohibited today. In fact, the only items that would appear on a list today are coffee, wine, beer, and nuts for the child less than 3 years of age. Nuts should be avoided because of the possible danger of choking, not for nutritional reasons.

By 2 years of age, children should be eating three meals per day with snacks in mid-morning and mid-afternoon if the snacks do not suppress the mealtime appetite. Vitamin supplements are not recommended for use by children unless the child has a special nutritional requirement or recognized vitamin deficiency.

QUESTIONS FOR THE MOTHER ABOUT CHAPTER 8

1. Why has a child's diet more to do with its future welfare than any other thing?

1910 The correct diet of a baby and child is responsible for the bone, teeth, muscle, physical reserve, mental capacity that is needed by a successful adult. The following bills of fare for young children were prepared by Dr. Charles V. Chapin, Commissioner of Health, Providence, R.I., May 1909. [The menus included in the original chapter are omitted because they are much more specific than the advice given by physicians today.]

REFERENCE

1. American Academy of Pediatrics, Committee on Nutrition. *Pediatric Nutrition Handbook,* 2nd ed. Elk Grove Village, Illinois. 1985.

9
What You Ought to Know About Your School

The German doctors have invented the term "school sickness" to describe a malady which is even more wide-spread, I fear, in the New World, than in Germany. It is the direct product of the ancient pedagogical doctrine, that the more a child is forced to study, the more it will learn. A healthy youngster, exposed for a few years to the operations of this doctrine, is converted into a weak, sickly and inefficient being, with ragged nerves and a bad stomach. Its mind, perhaps, has acquired a mastery of the scale of G minor and of many irregular verbs, but its blood has forgotten how to grapple with germs.

The schoolmarm, like the loving mother, is too assiduous in her attentions. The mother, coddling her child, measurably increases its chances of death (as I have shown in past chapters); and the teacher, seeking to lead it too precipitately into the Elysian fields of knowledge, sadly over-burdens its brain and its eyes, its lungs and its muscles, its back and its nerves. The result of this classroom forcing is entirely and inevitably pernicious. No good can possibly come of it.

The teacher, I suppose, is really not to blame, after all, for if the mother were not behind her egging her on to her sinister task, she would probably let indolence serve the benevolent purpose of mercy. As it is, she is expected to convert the baby of four or five years into a virtuoso with an extensive repertoire of kindergarten arias; and by the time the poor child is seven, she must have instilled into it a comprehensive grasp of spelling, arithmetic, reading, writing, Mexican bead-work and plain sewing. The mother of such a prodigy is proud of its attainments, and feels a glow when bored friends hypocritically marvel. Later on she will wonder why her child has watery eyes, constant colds or round shoulders.

As a matter of fact, it seems to me to be very unwise to send a boy or girl to school until the age of eight, at least. In America, six is the common age for beginning with the three R's, and four and a half the age for kindergarten mummery, but it is entirely improbable that this early start is an advantage, even if the mere accumulation of knowledge be accepted as the sole aim of education. It is beginning to be recognized more that the child which begins school at eight is far more capable of learning quickly than the child which begins at six; and at ten the former is almost certain to know as much as the latter, despite the fact that one has had four years of schooling, while the other has had but half as much. And after that, there will begin to appear a noticeable difference between the two. The one will bear some permanent mark of its too-early bending over desk and slate; the other will be a healthy animal.

The healthy boy of six displays little or no inclination to dally with books. His thirst for knowledge is satisfied by the accumulation of a vast store of baseball lore, with many intricate subtleties of rule, precedent and decision; and his natural yearning to be up and doing finds its proper outlet in purely physical activity. He eats plain, wholesome food, and he spends at least ten hours of the twenty-four in sleep. Between meals he is in the open air, galloping, marauding and fighting his fellows. He is a savage, true-enough—but that touch of savagery will be worth more to him than Greek in the years to come, when he is a grown man doing the hard work of the world, and needs an abounding reserve of brute vigor to draw upon.

Against this tough and uncultivated boy place the typical young pundit of his years. This last is a master, not only of the spelling-book, but also of the works of Oliver Optic.* He is studious and his parents are proud of him. Instead of chasing three-baggers in the outfield, he traces the course of the river Amazon. He is quiet, reserved, polite, obedient—and has a touch of mild vanity. He has no liking for the barbarous sports of other boys. He excels at none of their games. At a baseball match he is content to keep score.

---

*Oliver Optic was the pseudonym of William Taylor Adams (1822–1897), the author of over 100 books for children.

Such a boy I believe, is as abnormal as a boy with an obvious physical deformity. Instead of being encouraged in his unhealthy studiousness, as is commonly the case, he should be taken from school and, to borrow a lowly term, "turned out to grass." That is to say, he should be led, willy-nilly, into the savage mode of life of the normal boy, in the hope that it will awaken in him some spark of the savage. His dislike for games is really nothing but a feeling of physical incapacity. He realizes that he is not as strong and tough as other boys, and so he shrinks from competing with them. Let him put his books aside for a while—let him straighten up his bent back, breathe pure air, get wet by the rain, and make acquaintance with splinters, bruises and sunburn—and his shrinking will begin to disappear. Some day, let us hope, he will have progressed so far that he will return home with a black eye, acquired honorably in open and valiant combat. When that day arrives, it will be time to send him back to school.

Three hours a day is enough study for any child during its first year or two in school, and this period should be broken by a recess of at least half an hour. In many large American cities the day's session is divided into two parts—one of two and a half or three hours and the other of two hours or less, with an intermission of an hour or an hour and a half. This is rather too much for the child of seven or eight, especially since home study is commonly added, but there is one saving grace to the scheme, and that lies in the long midday recess.

It is very important that the meal eaten during this recess be a warm one, and whenever possible it should be prepared and eaten at home. Until a child is ten or twelve years old it must have its dinner, or principal meal of the day, at noon. The rest of the household may dine in the evening, but for the youngster so heavy a repast near bedtime is certain to be deleterious. A bundle of cold sandwiches will not serve as a substitute for the midday dinner, for the child needs not only the warm, home-cooked food, but also the walk home, the change of scene, the bit of play on the way, and the hour's forgetfulness of lessons.

Sitting still for two or three hours is an exhausting and painful proceeding to a child of seven or eight. It is as painful, almost, as it would be for a grown man to stand immovable for the same length of time. The child, unable to bear the strain, is apt to lounge in some unhealthful manner. Out of this lounging—this resting upon the desk—come round shoulders. And out of round shoulders come a host of ills.

The strain upon the back, in school, is equaled by the tax upon the eyes. If blackboards were really black, they might justify their existence, but in practice they are usually a dirty gray, which reflects the light in blinding flashes and subjects the eyes to harassing duty. From them the child turns to its book—and there it encounters more assaults upon its vision. The fruits of this eye-strain are so many that it would be impossible to catalogue them. They range from irritability and headache to serious derangements of the digestion.

How many mothers who read this have ever entered the schoolrooms in which their children spend from four to six hours a day? It is not common, I believe, for such visits of inspection to be made, and in many places they are no doubt discouraged by the pedagogic authorities, but they are plainly a part of every mother's duty. You may find that your child is forced to sit all day beside a drafty window or near a heater; that it is so far from the blackboard that it can scarcely see; that it occupies a desk too large or too small for it; or that its schoolroom is a dark, evil-smelling, ill-ventilated place.

Suppose one or another of these conditions is found? What can you do to remedy it? Well, you can protest, certainly, and if your single protest does no good you can get other mothers to protest with you. If the school is a private one, and you are paying tuition, your objections will be heard politely enough; and even if it is a public school, and the principal is entrenched behind the patronage of the ward boss, you will not find him so independent as you may think. The disgusting condition of the public schools in many American cities is due almost entirely to the lethargy of parents. Whenever and wherever there has been intelligent and active criticism of school methods and housing, substantial reforms have followed. Even a ward boss has a healthy respect for the collective indignation of a party of mothers.

If, after exerting your best efforts to work improvements, you find that alarming conditions still exist, take your child away from school, by all means—especially if it is still under nine years old. It is during the first few years that the greatest damage is done, and the least advantage gained by risking it. I am firmly convinced, indeed, that the average school does more harm than good to all children under nine. Too many are herded into one class, and too little attention is paid to individual idiosyncrasies. The theory is that all children of an age are alike—a theory comparable, for soundness, to the political doctrine that all men are equally capable of voting intelligently. The bright child is retarded by the stupid ones, and the healthy child is contaminated by the unhealthy child. The level that is thus attained is a very low level, indeed.

No doubt there has occurred to many readers a practical objection to one part of my argument. It is this: that if a child be kept from school until it is eight years old it will go through its whole period of schooling two years behind the child which began at six. The children in a school are not taught individually, but in classes, and after it is once entered in a class, a child's rate of progress is the class rate of progress.

In answer to this, let me suggest that the child be kept from school, not only until it is eight, but until it is ten. Let it spend its whole time at play until it is eight, and then let it begin to study at home, either under its mother's supervision or in care of some competent teacher. If it begins with two hours a day, and proceeds to three and finally four, it will be fully as far advanced, after two years, as the child which has spent four years picking up a haphazard knowledge of the rudiments in the average schoolroom. It will then be possible to enter, not in the first class, but in the fifth, and it will go through the succeeding classes with children of its age.

The labor of teaching a child the things taught in the first few grades of a primary school is not nearly so forbidding as you may imagine. In the classroom the individual child gets no more than a few minutes of the teacher's undivided attention a day, and yet it makes progress. If you fancy that it derives much benefit from the instruction given to the other children, you have but to visit a classroom to be undeceived. On the contrary, most of its time, when it is not actually performing its own day's task, is spent in necessary, if unlawful, efforts to relieve the intolerable tedium of its imprisonment.

I am convinced, indeed, that an ordinarily intelligent child, with an hour's individual instruction a day, five days a week, can make far greater progress than the average child in the average classroom. And just consider what it gains! Instead of being shut up for hours in a noisy room, it has one hour of work and all the rest of its time for play—for fresh-air and healthful muscular activity. If it arises moody or dull, its hour of study may be removed from morning to afternoon, or divided into two half hours. It may devote the whole of the rare, bright days of Winter to play, and make up for its lost time on stormy days. It will have a clean, airy room for study, with no distractions; warm meals; and no home-study tasks for the evening.

Later on, of course, the school will begin to reckon—if only for the salutary effect that its rough democracy and emulation have upon character. But for the very young child the classroom holds out few advantages. It is the easiest way, perhaps, but it is always the way of headache, anemia, lassitude, nervousness, hysteria and broken health.

Commentary

Chapter 9: What You Ought to Know About Your School

Although most of the opinions presented in this essay are based on little fact and much bravado, the inclusion of a discussion on schools and school-related problems seems particularly prescient on the authors' part. The subject was not given much attention by pediatricians of the era, perhaps because of the preoccupation with issues such as infant feeding and infectious diseases. For example, neither Dr. L. Emmett Holt's 1174-page textbook of pediatrics nor his best selling primer, *The Care and Feeding of Children,* ventured to comment upon the medical or psychological implications of an institution that occupied 33% of the average child's daily life. Other textbooks of pediatrics published between 1890 and 1910 also generally ignored the topic.[1]

Yet as the century progressed the effect of schools on a child's life and health could not help but become an important issue to those who care for children. Coinciding with the rise of the public health movement, the institution of mass public school education in America began in the mid-19th century.[2] As the nation's population grew and more children enrolled in public schools, overcrowding and underfinancing of the schools became acute problems. Several school systems across the country simply lacked the funds, buildings, or facilities to provide good education for the burgeoning number of pupils. Many schools from the 1890s well into the 1910s conducted classes in poorly lit and underventilated basements, corridors, and temporary wooden structures called "portables." Inadequate plumbing and sewage systems meant that classrooms were often filled with the stench of poorly working toilets or overfilled outhouses, which must have impeded the zest for learning. These deplorable conditions prompted Mencken to urge parents to protest in order to effect a change for the better.

School Inspections

Many physicians became interested in the interactions between school and health in order to help prevent or control the outbreaks of infectious diseases such as diphtheria, scarlet fever, and measles. For example, in 1893 the city of New York appointed the nation's first school medical inspector, Dr. Moreau Morse, for exactly such a purpose.[3] Two years later, the city of Boston organized the first system of school medical inspection and appointed 50 physicians under the direction of Dr. Samuel Durgin to oversee the health care needs of its 50 school districts.[4,5] A program of school inspections, which had been in operation in Europe since the 1830s, soon caught on in other states, and by 1915 there was a large body of legislation pertaining to health inspection in schools. Such legislation provided for the funding of physicians to make frequent visits to the schools of a particular district and to examine children singled out by teachers, visiting nurses, or fellow students for evidence of illness.

Medical inspection of the schools in the United States continued to expand during the second decade of the 20th century. Individual schools were staffed with full-time nurses, organized plans were outlined for the isolation of children suspected of having a contagious disease, and vision and hearing examinations were provided. Doctors offered medical consultations for the diagnosis and therapy of illnesses or physical defects other than infectious diseases, school buildings were inspected to ensure sound measures of sanitation and safety, and classes in hygiene were offered to teachers, parents, and students. Soon other professionals became interested in the fields of school hygiene and occupational health. Engineers published widely on better means of lighting and ventilating school buildings, the provision of adequate plumbing systems, desks designed for children, blackboards that would not promote eye strain, and other relevant considerations. Architects began to consider the issue of safety in the design of school buildings. And educators were faced with the task of coordinating the diverse efforts of the many factions who wished to improve the public school system.[6,7] Finally, parents who had read about the school hygiene movement in the popular press or had concerns about their children's health became school health advocates as well.

Mencken and Hirshberg were undoubtedly aware of the public's interest in the schools when they decided to include this essay in *The Delineator* series. In fact, over 500 articles on school hygiene had appeared in print in the medical literature and popular periodicals between 1908 and 1909.[8] School hygiene was a "hot topic." Yet the original outline for the baby articles submitted by Mencken to Dreiser in 1908 dealt exclusively with health issues of the infant. There survives no mention about an essay on schools. One can only speculate that the increasing attention to school hygiene in both the medical and lay press prompted discussion of the subject. The resulting essay is a distinctly Menckenian discourse on Mencken's perceptions of the flaws in the educational system, a topic that interested him and inspired many opinionated and bombastic diatribes throughout his career.

Mencken's School Days

Mencken had unhappy memories of his days at the F. Knapp Institute, a private elementary school "that catered to the boys and girls of the Baltimore bourgeoisie for more than 60 years."[9] Although he was valedictorian of his high school class at the Baltimore Polytechnic Institute in 1896, his aversion to formal education lasted throughout his adult life. Mencken rejected his father's offer to send him to college, and announced that he wanted to write and see the world as a newspaperman. He often proclaimed the superiority of his self-motivated style of education—learning from a "front row seat" to the world—over the dull, stagnant classrooms conducted in colleges by "chalky pedagogues." And although it is pure speculation, it might be that Mencken's vociferous prejudice against formal education was a means of justifying his own lack of it. If learning and becoming an educated man from independent reading, writing, and observing the world at large were good enough for the Sage of Baltimore, it should be good enough for everyone else. For example, Mencken published an essay in 1918 denigrating the "professional teacher" who was more preoccupied with the techniques of teaching than with the subject matter.[10] He preferred listening to and learning from the intelligent man who had a love and enthusiasm for the subject he taught over the entire lot of self-touting, overinflated pedagogues. In a 1928 newspaper column, Mencken referred to school days as follows:

> ...the unhappiest in the whole span of human existence. They are full of dull unintelligible tasks, new and unpleasant ordinances, brutal violations of common sense and common decency. It doesn't take a reasonably bright boy long to discover that most of what is rammed into him is nonsense, and that no one really cares very much whether he learns it or not. His parents, unless they are infantile in mind, tend to be bored by his lessons and labors, and are unable to conceal the fact from his sharp eyes. His first teachers he views simply as disagreeable policemen. His later ones he usually sets down quite accurately as asses.[11]

"What You Ought to Know About Your Schools" is consistent with Mencken's strong bias against formal education. It is of particular interest to the Mencken reader because it predates his better known anti-pedagogy essays. Trying to explain Mencken's arcane opinions on how long a school day should be or what type of activities should occupy a child's day would serve no purpose. Instead, we shall let the essay speak for itself and clarify two points Mencken makes on "school sickness" and the importance of recess.

School Sickness

Mencken describes a vague and dubious malady called "school sickness" that is caused by the overzealous teacher who overworks his or her students into fits of exhaustion. Despite Mencken's sensational and graphic prose, however, there is no reason to believe that too much concentration on the "mastery of the scale of G minor and of many irregular verbs" causes the blood to lose its ability to "grapple with germs." Good health rests upon the foundations of a balanced diet, adequate sleep, and physical exercise, and a reasonably rigorous education does not, in itself, make a child more susceptible to illness.

The style of education Mencken refers to, where students slaved away for hours at rote memorization never to see the light of day, probably had its origins in 17th century Germany. During the complex and disruptive Thirty Year War (1618–1648), Emperor Ferdinand II, the Catholic monarch of the German Empire, seized control of Bohemia and rescinded all of the reforms of its Calvinist ruler, Frederick V. Among these included Ferdinand's placement of all educational institutions under the control of the Jesuit Order of the Catholic Church. The Jesuits' strict style of education, which was characterized by rote memorization and corporal punishment, set a precedent for the demanding, systematic, no-nonsense style of the German classroom for the next 200 years.[12] Opponents to this method of education felt that too much emphasis was placed upon the memorization of facts and not enough attention was paid to the development of one's body. The children enrolled in such a system obviously were also unhappy and were, reportedly, unenthusiastic about their studies, often listless, and frequently ill.[13] School sickness emerged as a concept to explain why so many German pupils were "sickly" and susceptible to infectious diseases. However, the proponents of the theory that arduous education caused illness failed to take into account other important contributing factors such as poor nutrition and hygiene, the types and virulence of infectious organisms prevalent at the time, and, possibly, an entity pediatricians now call "school phobia"—a child avoids going to school by complaining of any number of vague symptoms that resemble illness (e.g., headaches, stomach aches, sore throats, etc.).

Recess

The importance of recess and physical activity as part of the school curriculum is emphasized, although ironically Mencken hated physical activity even as a child and avoided it whenever possible. He was "round shouldered" and wore a brace to correct the deformity. He was consistently beaten in games and fights with his younger brother, Charlie. Indeed, his description of a boy who "instead of chasing three-baggers in the outfield" would rather trace "the course of the river Amazon" seems painfully autobiographical. Nevertheless, Mencken's dislike for physical activity failed to make him "sickly" and he was rarely ill until his late teens, when he probably contracted tuberculosis, which remained quiescent throughout his life.

Recess was first introduced into the school curriculum in 1418 by the Italian schoolmaster and rhetoritician Vittorino de Feltre.[14] Vittorino insisted that equal attention be given to the teaching of hygiene and physical education, in addition to formal subjects, at his school in Mantua. He devised programs of exercise and advocated various forms of free play after noting that children were more eager to learn and more successful with their studies if periods of free play and physical activity were interspersed with didactic sessions. Recess was removed from the school curriculum in Germany, coinciding with the institution of Jesuit education in Bohemia in the early 17th century. It was only begrudgingly reinstituted by German schools in the late 1800s. Few educators or physicians today would disagree with Mencken's contention that the school day needs to be broken up with periods of play in order to promote the development of physical fitness and to add an element of fun to the school experience.

QUESTIONS FOR THE MOTHER ABOUT CHAPTER 9

1. Why do you send your child to school?

1910 To fit him for life—to make him a self-supporting, self-respecting, happy citizen. What is the first essential to this—good health—with it nine-tenths of the battle of life are won.

Current To obtain an education and to learn to socialize with others.

2. What are the years when health is established?

1910 From birth to 16 years of age.

Current Good health and good health practices are established during the first two decades of life. Maintenance of healthy practices then becomes the challenge for the remainder of life.

3. How many of these years are spent in school?

1910 Ten or eleven.

Current Formal education today, for the child who does not go to college or graduate school, is 13 years.

4. Could an unheathful school environment unfit a child for life?

1910 Yes, it often does.

Current Yes.

5. How?

1910 Bad air breeds contagion. Bad air and contagious diseases undermine a child's vitality—poor light, dirty windows, shiny blackboards, fine print, glossy paper, too much close-range work strain a child's eyes. Eye-strain causes indigestion, nervousness, injured eyesight. Ill-adjusted desks cause round shoulders, curved spines, restlessness. Too little recess—relaxation from application to lessons—overstrains the child's nerves and disgusts him with school work or any work.

Dust, dry-sweeping, unclean rooms spread tuberculosis—sun, fresh air, soap and disinfectant kill tuberculosis germs.

Cold lunch eaten at school gives a child indigestion—malnutrition. Every child should have a hot, hearty, nourishing dinner, at noon, *at home if possible.*

Current By exposing the child unnecessarily to infectious agents and environmental toxins, such as asbestos, and by failing to teach basic health essentials such as how to eat properly, how to avoid sexually transmitted diseases, and the dangers of illicit drugs, alcohol, and smoking.

6. Should not the place where your child spends the greater part of his days for at least 9 months in the year receive every mother's individual attention?

1910 By all means. Neglect of the school environment might mean life-long failure to the child and disappointment to the mother and father.

Current Yes, but it should receive every mother *and father's* attention.

7. What should a mother look for in her child's school?

1910 Open windows, a schoolroom thermometer, adjustable desks *adjusted*—clean floors—scrubbed—*not dry swept*—good light for every child in the room—recess *out-of-doors*—individual drinking cups, individual towels.

Cleanly dressed children.

A medical inspector to examine the children for contagious diseases—such as consumption, measles, scarlet fever, pneumonia, diphtheria, mumps, colds, sore throats, tonsillitis, scabies, pediculosis. A physician to examine children for physical defects such as bad teeth, adenoids, enlarged tonsils, defects of hearing and sight, tuberculosis.

Current Parents should examine the curriculum as well as the physical plant and the medical facilities. Classrooms and bathrooms should be clean, well lighted, and well ventilated. The cafeteria and the kitchen should be examined. The qualifications of the nurse and the procedures followed when a child is sick should be reviewed.

8. Are these things absolutely essential to the good health of school children?
1910 Yes.
Current Yes.

9. What should a mother do if she finds these essentials lacking?
1910 She should go to the principal of the school and ask to have defects of school equipment rectified. If the principal cannot do this she should go to the school board and make complaint. If the school board will or can do nothing, she should put the matter before the citizens of her town, either through the local paper, Mothers' Club or Citizens' Union. No government can long resist the demands of a number of parents for the welfare of their children.
Current Bring problems to the attention of the school principal first. If the principal takes no action, then complaints should be brought to the Parent-Teacher's Association (PTA), then the Superintendent of Schools and the local Board of Education.

10. What should a mother do if the school doctor finds physical defects in her child?
1910 She should at once send the child to a physician, dentist, or surgeon and have the defect rectified. If taken in time the child can usually be made normal. If neglected its health will be undermined.
Current Promptly have physical problems or disorders evaluated by the child's own physician or local hospital department of pediatrics. Persist in this course until the matter is resolved.

11. Should children with tuberculosis be allowed to be in school with other children?
1910 Never.
In some cities there are special schools for tuberculous children. It is not safe to risk infection of well children. It is very unfair to the tuberculous child. It needs fresh air all the time, very little mental effort, plenty of rest and sleep, large quantities of milk and eggs and the constant attention of a physician.

Current Only if the child is receiving medication and the disease has been shown not to be in the contagious stage. This is really not much of a problem in the United States today.

12. How can the tuberculous children be weeded out?

1910 Every child should be examined for tuberculosis before entering school each fall. Children with tuberculous parents should have special tests. Their sputum should be examined bacteriologically and tuberculin skin test made. Children who have not tuberculosis, but have tuberculous parents, or are especially weak, should be in school but part of the day; the rest of the day they should be out-of-doors or resting. They should have a feeding of milk and eggs between meals, morning and afternoon.

Current Most schools require a health examination before admission, and skin testing for tuberculosis may be part of the examination. Periodic health examinations are also performed in most schools, at which time a rare case of tuberculosis might be identified.

REFERENCES

1. See also Meigs JF, Pepper W. *A Practical Treatise on the Diseases of Children*, 7th ed., Philadelphia, 1882; and Rotch TM. *Pediatrics: The Medical and Hygienic Treatment of Children*, Philadelphia, 1896.
2. Duffy J. School vaccination: The precursor to school medical inspection. *Journal of the History of Medicine and Allied Sciences* 33:344–355, 1978.
3. Gulick LH, Ayres LP. *Medical Inspection of Schools*. New York: Russell Sage Foundation, 1909, pp. 18–28.
4. Sullivan JT, Murphy TJ, Cronin MJ. Medical inspection of the schools from the standpoint of the medical inspector. *Boston Medical and Surgical Journal* 159:815–820, 1908.
5. Coues WP. The medical inspection of schools in Boston: The present limitations and future possibilities. *Boston Medical and Surgical Journal* 160:746–748, 1909.
6. Gulick and Ayres, *Medical Inspection of Schools*, pp. 52–65, 66–103, 104–136, 137–149.
7. Young JE. Hygiene of the school age. In Abt IA (ed.): *Pediatrics*, Vol. 1. Philadelphia, W.B. Saunders, 1923, pp. 866–1131.
8. This figure was arrived at by tabulating all the articles listed under the headings "schools" or "school hygiene" for the years 1908 and 1909 in *Index Medicus* and the *Reader's Guide to Periodical Literature*.
9. Mencken HL. *Happy Days*. New York: Alfred A. Knopf, 1940, p. 20.
10. Mencken HL. The educational process. New York *Evening Mail* Jan. 23, 1918.

11. Mencken HL. Travail. Baltimore *Evening Sun* Oct. 8, 1928.

12. Durant W, Durant A. *The Age of Reason Begins*. New York: Simon & Schuster, 1961, pp. 555–558.

13. Burnham WH. *Great Teachers and Mental Health: A Study of Seven Educational Hygienists*. New York: D. Appleton and Co., 1926, p. 7.

14. Ibid., pp. 103–120.

10
Need Every Child Have "Catching Diseases?"

The notion that every child is doomed to suffer from *catching diseases* at some time during its first ten years is a dangerous and stupid error. There is no more reason why a child need have diphtheria, scarlet fever, measles, or whooping cough than why it need have smallpox, lockjaw or hydrophobia if proper preventive methods be used. All these infections are preventable.

Commentary

An Introduction to the Infectious and Communicable Diseases of Childhood

The rate of infant mortality in the United States has steadily declined as the 20th century has progressed, a result of numerous victories in the conquest of infectious diseases. The descriptions of the infectious diseases in the remaining chapters serve as a reminder that enormous progress has been made in eliminating the threats of many deadly illnesses. For example, in 1988 10 infants per 1000 died before 1 year of age; the major cause of death was complications from extreme prematurity. As Shakespeare's King Richard III lamented, "Deformed, unfinished, sent before my time into this breathing world scarce half made up."[1]

In 1910, between 150 and 200 infants per 1000 died before their first birthday. The culprits were almost exclusively infectious diseases. Indeed, the excellent health enjoyed by the majority of our nation's children today is mainly attributable to the successful prevention of poliomyelitis, tetanus, pertussis (whooping cough), measles, mumps, and rubella through vaccination programs, rehydration therapies for gastroenteritis and diarrhea, and the treatment of bacterial infections with antibiotics. The physicians in 1910 had little to offer acutely ill patients other than quarantines, which were believed to arrest the spread of contagious diseases, supportive measures such as bed rest and nourishing foods, folk remedies without any medicinal value, and a sympathetic demeanor. During a period when disorders such as diarrhea, gastroenteritis, diphtheria, pneumonia, scarlet fever, whooping cough, and measles were so closely associated with death, it is not unexpected that 40% of *What You Ought to Know About Your Baby* is devoted to the presentation and prevention of infectious diseases.

Humoralism and Disease

Before the scientific revolution of the late 19th century, when Robert Koch, Louis Pasteur, and others predicted and proved that many diseases were manifestations of infections caused by different microscopic organisms, none of the laboratory tests and technology we take for granted today was available to help confirm a difficult diagnosis. Physicians who practiced before the development and substantiation of the germ theory were frequently confused by the challenge of differentiating one disease from another. Matters became especially confusing when different diseases shared similar symptoms.

Beginning with the ancient Greeks and continuing well into the 1800s, doctors focused on the symptoms exhibited by their patients and explained them using the concept of *humoralism,* the belief that diseases were caused by an imbalance or abnormal mixture of what were thought to be the four major components, or humors, of the human body: blood, phlegm, yellow bile, and black bile. At a time when dissection was illegal and physicians had limited firsthand knowledge of the human body and its workings beyond the skin, important emphasis was placed on fluids that were expelled or excreted during an illness. For example, gastrointestinal diseases were believed to be due to an excess of black and yellow bile; cathartics, laxatives, and purgatives that emptied the bowels of these bad humors would have been prescribed. Cardiovascular diseases such as dropsy or congestive heart failure were thought to be caused by an excess of blood and the excess would be alleviated by bleeding the patient. Hence, a perceived surplus of a specific humor would yield an imbalance or disease. Intervention by a physician trained in humoralism was limited to removal of the offending bad humor and observation. This theory strongly influenced the perception of disease as being entirely of internal origin, disregarding the possibility that a factor or germ in the patient's environment could cause illness. The very idea that a disease might be caused by an invisible germ was laughable. So well regarded by physicians and natural philosophers was the concept of humoralism that it was practiced for over 17 centuries.[2]

Solidism

By the late 18th century, humoralism began to be intensely questioned. Scientists no longer believed its precepts to be valid and, instead, subscribed to a theory proposed by an Italian pathologist, Giovanni Morgagni. After years of careful dissection at the autopsy table, Morgagni described a number of specific lesions in various organs that he correlated to specific symptoms and illnesses displayed by living patients. The theory was called solidism and relied upon the tenet that form defines function.[3] Organs that had their original form changed in a specific manner would perform differently or aberrantly. Rudolf Virchow, the German pathologist, embraced these concepts in the early 19th century, using the description "the anatomical idea."

Virchow refined Morgagni's observations at the autopsy table by studying how organs and tissues changed microscopically in response to different stimuli and conditions. The pathologist and his graduate students were able to describe the seats of disease on a cellular level and proposed that diseases resulted from an imbalance in cells, explainable by the laws of physics or chemistry. Although the explanation for the cause of disease had changed from an imbalance of four specific fluids to alterations in function of the cells that make up the body, the anatomical idea still closely resembled the concept of humoralism — that illness is the result of an internal imbalance.

The Germ Theory

A new concept of disease, the germ theory, emerged as the 19th century progressed. Its proponents acknowledged that although many diseases do result from internal imbalances, many others are communicable and are caused by specific microscopic agents. By the 1890s, the germ theory had begun to gain support from bacteriologists, scientists, and eventually physicians and surgeons, and by the beginning of the 20th century, was considered fact for many infectious diseases. A major part of biomedical research during the years 1870 to 1930 focused on the search for the agents that caused contagious diseases. For example, Robert Koch isolated the dread tubercle bacillus that causes tuberculosis in 1882. From his work came the famed and rigid Koch's postulates for identifying pathogenic microbes: (1) the microbe must always be found in lesions of the disease it supposedly causes; (2) the microbe must be isolated in pure culture or growth on artificial medium; (3) if bacteria grown on an artificial medium were injected into an experimental animal, the animal would develop the illness; and (4) the organism in question must then be recovered from lesions in the experimental animal.[4] Only by satisfying each of these postulates could a bacteriologist claim that a specific organism caused a specific disease. Koch's postulates were the guiding scientific principles for Friedrich Loeffler in 1884 when he discovered the diphtheria bacillus, Jules Bordet and Octave Gengou who isolated pertussis in 1906, and Gladys and George Dick who established hemolytic streptococci as the cause of scarlet fever in 1923.

Bacteria, of course, are not the only microorganisms that cause childhood illness. A large variety of viruses may also attack children, and the 20th century has witnessed the elucidation of a number of viral illnesses, including measles, rubella, poliomyelitis, and influenza. And the war against infectious diseases is far from over. Even today, new or previously undetected contagious diseases continue to vex physicians; for example, Lyme disease, a form of arthritis caused by a bacteria passed to humans by ticks; cat-scratch disease, a form of generalized lymph node swelling and malaise caused by a bacteria passed from cats to humans; and, of course, the human immunodeficiency virus of acquired immune deficiency syndrome (AIDS).

Quarantine

Quarantines probably began as a community's response to a deadly, contagious disease. As though responding to an opposing army, the town threatened by an epidemic would shut its gates, refusing entry to outsiders or their goods. Medical historian David Musto defines the quarantine "as a legal demarcation between two groups intended to prevent the penetration of a biological contaminant into the unaffected group."[5]

The word quarantine literally means 40 days and referred to the period of time ships coming into the port of Venice were required to dock before their goods, passengers, and crew could disembark. Quarantines were probably first instituted in Venice during the 14th century in direct response to the Black Death, or bubonic plague, although lepers were physically separated and ostracized from society during biblical times and the early Middle Ages. The 40-day quarantine had nothing to do with the natural history, incubation period, or epidemiology of bubonic plague; physicians did not yet think about diseases in such terms or concepts. Instead, it was considered to be a long enough period to allow the epidemic to "burn itself out."

The cause of bubonic plague was unknown; it was a strikingly sudden illness manifested by extreme weakness, high fever, marked swelling of the lymph glands, and frequently death.[6] Most people during the 14th century believed that such pestilence was a punishment for sinners and a direct result of God's wrath.[7] Unfortunately, this misconception that one who contracts a horrible illness did something to deserve it was the leading explanation of disease for centuries. During the plague epidemic of the 1350s, separation or isolation of affected individuals was justified on the basis that the survival of the community was more important than the individual's right to function in society; quarantine also had religious overtones, i.e., to keep sinners separate from the healthy and righteous.

As medicine progressed, physicians began to appreciate the distinguishing characteristics and presentations of different infectious diseases. The type of quarantine imposed was adapted to the disease at hand. Frequently, however, quarantines failed to arrest the spread of a contagious disease, and it became clear that they were not the solution to the control of epidemics. For example, the years 1832, 1849, and 1866 were notable for major cholera epidemics in the United States. Cholera is an infectious form of profuse diarrhea; the patient also experiences severe vomiting, abdominal cramps, dehydration, and, before the advent of intravenous rehydration therapy, death. In order for cholera to manifest itself, the bacteria that causes it, *Vibrio comma* (a name used because of the organism's shape), must find its way into the victim's gastrointestinal tract, i.e., the victim must ingest something contaminated with *Vibrio comma*. Cholera is thus spread primarily through contaminated water and foods. Isolating individuals with cholera but neglecting to clean up the infected city's water supply or food chain is ineffective. Such misapplication of the quarantine only serves to restrict the individual's freedom without any real benefit to disease control. The quarantine is probably only reasonably instituted for a disease that is transmitted by casual person-to-person contact and that threatens the safety of the public at large. It was usually misapplied to outbreaks based not on medical principles but rather upon fear of the disease in question. Using the example of the cholera epidemic of 1832, in New York City a quarantine was instituted against the entry of ships and vehicles; this quarantine was mandated by the public and the mayor of New York, despite advice to the contrary by the medical community that it would not work.[8] It did not.

There were diseases such as tuberculosis, for which quarantine was somewhat more useful in checking the spread of an infection. Tuberculosis could be contracted merely by conversing with an infected person, particularly if the carrier coughed and the victim inhaled expelled tubercle bacilli. Physical separation of persons with tuberculosis until their disease became quiescent or inactive was considered by many experts during the early 20th century to be the only means of halting its spread, although the practice did little to cure or treat the disease. Public health authorities and physicians held that the public's safety outweighed the individual's rights, and state legislatures across the nation responded by enacting mandatory tuberculosis testing, reporting to the board of health those who tested "positive," and requiring admission (separation) of affected individuals to a tuberculosis hospital or sanitarium. TB sanitariums disappeared with the development of antituberculosis drugs in the 1950s.

Today it is not uncommon to hear discussions of why past precedents of quarantining and isolating persons with tuberculosis and other infectious diseases cannot be applied to AIDS patients and people who have tested positive for the AIDS virus antibody. Most authorities believe that the use of quarantine would be ill-advised and practically useless because transmission of the disease is anything but casual and rarely accidental, even in health care workers. Indeed, a recently published chapter on the latter subject begins, "HIV [the AIDS virus] is one of the least transmissible occupational pathogens."[9]

Nevertheless, the discussion of the proper management of the AIDS epidemic continues to be an ethical and moral see-saw between the private rights of affected individuals and society's demand for safety. The situation is certainly in flux, but one would hope that measures such as mandatory testing for HIV status, required reporting to Boards of Public Health, and contact tracing are carefully studied to ascertain efficacy before they are implemented on a full-scale basis. Public disclosure of the identity of an AIDS patient can result in harsh indignities directly as a result of discriminatory and other ignorant practices, and therefore those who have responsibility for public health have a duty to require that all methods or plans to control the AIDS epidemic be proven safe and effective for all concerned before they are approved.

Similar to the contemporary dilemma surrounding AIDS, Mencken and Hirshberg had no vaccines to offer. They could only offer advice on good nursing care and avoidance of contact with a person known to have a contagious disease. Today the diseases Mencken and Hirshberg described are either largely preventable with immunizations or treatable with medications, rendering obsolete much of the discussion about disinfecting the sick room or quarantining a patient. However, the essays are of historical and literary interest. The description of the pathology of pneumonia and the explanation of how diphtheria antitoxin is produced and administered are engaging and informative. Mencken skillfully serves factual material in palatable prose on the unfelicitous topics of diphtheria, scarlet fever, whooping cough, pneumonia, and measles. Also, in view of the misinformation surrounding the AIDS epidemic today, the management of equally deadly diseases in the early 1900s without the benefit of today's medical technology is instructive.

The question and answer sections at the end of this chapter and the ones on diphtheria, whooping cough, pneumonia, and measles have been reprinted without being updated because they are not relevant to today's practice of medicine.

QUESTIONS FOR THE MOTHER ABOUT CHAPTER 10

1. What is the best method for the prevention of contagious diseases?

1910 Thorough physical examination of the child at frequent intervals; a healthy condition of mouth and teeth; removal of enlarged tonsils or adenoid growths; care and isolation of a child with a cold or sore throat; living and sleeping in the fresh air.

2. Why do bad teeth, failure to brush teeth daily, neglected tonsils and adenoids favor contagious diseases?

1910 Because germs lodge in decayed teeth and in the unhealthy tissue of tonsils and adenoids.

3. Why does neglect of colds increase contagious diseases?

1910 Because a cold is often the first sign of such diseases as whooping cough, measles, scarlet fever, etc., at the time when these diseases are most infectious. Because a neglected cold may often result in pneumonia or tuberculosis.

4. What are the first steps to take when a child comes down with a contagious disease?

1910 Send for a doctor. Put the child to bed in a well-aired, sunny room. Keep it away from other members of the family. Keep persons who have been exposed to the disease away from other people or school. Report the disease to the Board of Health; put a notice on the door stating that the disease is present in the house.

5. What is the invariable treatment for contagious diseases?
1910
1. Fresh air.
2. Complete quarantine.
3. Disinfection of all sheets, dishes, clothing used for the patient.
4. Fumigation of the room.
5. Thorough examination of the child by a physician on recovery to prevent further complications.
6. Nourishing food, such as fresh eggs and milk, outdoor life and rest.

6. What should your medicine chest contain?

1910 Absorbent cotton, aseptic gauze, carbolic Vaseline, castor oil, hot water bag, and NO PATENT MEDICINES.

REFERENCES

1. Shakespeare W. *Richard III* (act I, scene i) *The Complete Works of William Shakespeare*. New York: Avenel Books, 1975. p. 627.
2. An excellent discussion on the theories of humoralism and solidism can be found in English PC. Diphtheria and theories of infectious disease. *Pediatrics* 76:1–9, 1985.
3. Morgagni GB. *The Seats and Causes of Diseases* (translated by B. Alexander) Birmingham, AL: The Classics of Medicine Library. 1983.
4. Davis BD, Dulbecco R, Eisen HN, Ginsberg HS. *Microbiology* (3rd ed.). Philadelphia, Harper and Row, 1980, p. 7.
5. Musto DF. AIDS and panic: enemies within. *The Wall Street Journal* April 28, 1987.
6. Calvert WJ. Plague. *In* Osler W. (ed.). *Osler's System of Medicine,* Vol. II. Philadelphia: Lea Brothers and Co., 1907, p. 762.
7. Rosen G. *A History of Public Health.* New York: MD Publications, 1958, p. 62–65.
8. Rosenberg CE. *The Cholera Years. The United States in 1832, 1849 and 1866.* Chicago: University of Chicago Press, 1962, pp. 1–9; 79–81.
9. Gerberding JL. Occupational HIV transmission: risk reduction. *In* Becker CE (ed.). *Occupational HIV Infection: Risks and Risk Reduction.* Occupational Medicine: State of the Art Reviews. Philadelphia: Hanley & Belfus, Inc., 1989. 4 (Special Issue): 21–24.

11
If Your Baby Had Diphtheria

Of all the maladies that afflict small children none causes more terror to the agonized mother than diphtheria. It has an air of mystery and awfulness. It seems, almost, to presage certain death. The doctor's reluctant verdict—his brief, but positive orders regarding isolation and nursing—the mention of antitoxin, of antiseptics, of subcutaneous injections—the posting of the warning sign upon the door—all of these things bring the mother of the little patient to a pitiable state of alarm.

And yet, for all its indubitable dangers, diphtheria is one of the diseases that modern medicine may fairly claim to have conquered. Its cause is known and its course is known. It may be prevented, and in the great majority of cases it may be cured. When the doctor pronounces its dread name, there is no reason whatever why one should give thought to grievous possibilities, because these possibilities, fortunately for the human race, are now happily remote. Ten years ago more than half of the babies who took diphtheria died from it. To-day the death-rate is less than one-tenth, and, under conditions easily attainable, than less one-twentieth.

The credit for this belongs absolutely to the men who devised and perfected diphtheria antitoxin. No other single medical discovery of recent years has better proved its value to the human race, or better justified the bold experimentation—the ruthless slaughter of rabbits and guinea pigs—the patient toil with culture tube and microscope—of medical science.

No doubt you have heard assertive persons say that antitoxin is a snare, and that it kills more babies than it cures, and perhaps this sort of criticism has made some impression upon you. If it has, be warned in time. Your own child may take diphtheria tomorrow. If it does, antitoxin is the only thing under the sun that will aid it. When your doctor tells you so, show your faith in him by letting him go ahead with his work of inoculation. Half an hour's delay means regret poignant and everlasting.

To understand the nature of diphtheria antitoxin it is necessary first of all, to know something about diphtheria. In the view of the layman it appears as an extraordinarily violent species of sore throat, with an unaccountable tendency to infect others and to end in death. In the view of the pathologist it is an acute infectious disease of the first class, caused by a definite organism called the *bacillus diphtheria,* which secretes a powerful soluble toxin, or poison; which, in turn, produces death by inhibiting the proper action of the heart.

The *bacillus diphtheria,* despite the popular notion of bacilli, is not an animal, but a plant. Unlike the varieties of vegetation that are most familiar to us, it does not need an immovable soil for its roots, but floats about and grows luxuriantly in the human blood, or in any other suitable liquid. It is so small that a microscope magnifying one thousand times barely reveals it. In shape it resembles a minute rod, rather thick in section, and with one end swelling out a bit. It tends to grow in curious little clusters which much resemble the five outstretched fingers of a human hand.

The *bacillus diphtheria* is very tenacious of life, and even when dried and seemingly withered, it is capable of remaining alive for months. This explains the fact that it is very difficult to stamp out an epidemic of diphtheria. Once the bacilli gain a foothold in a house, a school or a neighborhood, they are very apt to infect child after child. They float about in the air; they appear, in countless millions, in the mouths of children who are ill with the disease; and they appear, too, though in less number, in the mouths of those who may be perfectly well. Only the most skillful use of antiseptics, by some one with sound scientific knowledge, is of any value in the effort to stamp them out.

When a swarm of these bacilli takes lodgment in a child's throat or tonsils, they begin at once to increase and multiply. Within a few hours they are present by the billion. Each individual throws off a minute stream of poison, and these streams, commingling, attack the throat tissue. They kill the mucous membrane, and the little blood vessels below it rush scar-forming materials to the scene to repair the damage. At the same time the white blood corpuscles in the blood vessels engage the bacilli in combat—attacking them and trying to swallow them. Before long the scene of the battle is littered with all sorts of débris—dead membrane, dead bacilli, dead corpuscles, and bits of scar tissue. This débris, in the end, forms quite a large mass, and becomes, in fact, the familiar diphtheria throat membrane.

The membrane obstructs the windpipe of the sufferer, and unless something is done to break it strangulation is apt to follow. Sometimes it is necessary to cut into the neck of the patient below the place of obstruction and insert a silver tube, to give the lungs air. More often, it is possible to force a tube down the throat, in front of the membrane. This operation requires great skill, and should be entrusted only to some expert who has done it often before.

Despite the size and toughness of the membrane, however, strangulation is seldom the cause of death in diphtheria. Much more often, the patient dies of heart failure, produced by the activity of the poisons secreted by the bacilli. These poisons are frightfully virulent, and being soluble they are carried to all parts of the body in the blood stream. It is evident, therefore, that if they can be attacked and destroyed in the blood their power of doing damage may be broken. This office of attacking and destroying them is the function of diphtheria antitoxin.

The manufacture of the antitoxin is based upon the fact that healthy blood, whenever germ poisons appear in it, begins automatically and at once to make antidotes for them. Inject a few drops of diphtheria poison into the veins of a healthy, full-grown man, and his blood will at once neutralize it, and as a result he will show no bad effects whatever. If the amount injected be very small, his blood, indeed, will manufacture a great deal more antidote than is necessary to neutralize it, and will keep on making antidote for some time after all of the poison present has been rendered harmless.

But if a large quantity of poison be injected, or if active bacilli in large numbers are lodged somewhere in the body, and are hard at work sending forth more poison, the blood will soon give up the hopeless struggle. It will fight valiantly as long as possible, and in the course of the battle it will neutralize a vast quantity of poison, but in the end the enemy will be too strong for it, and it will surrender. This is what happens when a child is infected with diphtheria and a colony of bacilli lodge in its throat. For a while its blood fights on, but in the end it is overcome, and the poison begins to course, without obstruction, through its veins.

Fortunately, it is possible to lend the body aid by reinforcing it. And how? Simply by injecting into the patient's veins blood from some animal which is capable of making a better fight against diphtheria than a human being. In practice the animal selected is always the horse. It is a hardy, cleanly and healthy beast; it is capable of losing a great deal of blood without damage; and its blood has a peculiar capacity for opposing and neutralizing the poisons of the diphtheria bacillus.

A fine, strong horse is selected, and the manufacture of antitoxin is begun by injecting into one of its veins a small amount of diphtheria poison. The amount is so small that the blood of the horse neutralizes it at once, and the animal suffers no ill effects at all. Four days later twice as much poison is injected. This, too, is neutralized by the horse's blood, and in addition, the blood, stimulated to activity, manufactures a large extra portion of antidote. Four days later a still larger dose of poison is administered, and thereafter for six months the process is kept up. The horse's blood, in the long battle, always manages to keep a bit ahead of the poison. At the end of six months, it is so heavy with antidote that it is capable of neutralizing any conceivable amount of poison. The horse, in fact, is utterly diphtheria-proof. One might inject into its veins enough diphtheria poison to kill an army, and it would go unscathed.

All that remains is to draw off some of this immunized blood and get it into the veins of the human patient. The process, it is obvious, is a very simple one. One of the veins of the animal is opened, a quantity of its blood is collected, and a portion of this blood (after it has settled and has been strained) is injected into the human patient. The strained blood is a sticky, yellowish liquid. It is what the doctors and druggists call diphtheria antitoxin.

This antitoxin, then, is nothing more than horse blood which has acquired an extraordinary capacity for combating diphtheria poisons. When it enters the blood vessels of the patient it begins at once to seek out the diphtheria poisons and destroy them. It does its work almost instantaneously, and if enough is used, the result is certain. All of the diphtheria poisons are neutralized—and the patient begins to grow better.

But it is plain that the antitoxin must be used quickly and in sufficient quantity if this desirable end is to be achieved. So long as the patient's blood fights on unaided, the amount of poisons present in it will go on increasing. By and by these poisons may be present in such great quantity that they will begin to impede the action of the heart. When that stage is reached the patient is dying, and it is too late to battle with the disease.

Therefore, it is important that the diphtheria antitoxin be used just as soon as there is good ground for believing that diphtheria is present. If it is used on the first day of the disease, the latest statistics show that it will save the lives of ninety-eight patients out of one hundred. If its use is put off until the second day, it will save only ninety-six. If it is used after the fourth day, it will not save more than eighty out of a hundred.

And it must be used in sufficient quantity. If one injection does not bring relief, let there be another, and then another, and yet another. The antitoxin can do no harm. In cases on record, wherein its use has long been delayed, almost incredible quantities have been injected. The scientific physician has a safe rule. He knows that there is hope so long as life lasts; and so he proceeds with the treatment until the danger line is passed and the patient shows signs of it.

You mothers learn a great deal about the care of children, but in the presence of a disease as dangerous as diphtheria you must yield up the custody of your child to the doctor and the nurse. Your family doctor must be a man in whom you have implicit confidence. Select him with the utmost care, and do it, by preference, at some time when there is no sickness in the household. Then, after you have chosen him and sickness comes, give him the faith and support that his learning and experience deserve. His whole life is devoted to the cure of human ills, and your common sense will teach you that, if he is an intelligent man, this devotion must profit him in wide knowledge.

Do not oppose him or hamper him in the sick-room. He knows what is best for the patient. If he proposes to use antitoxin, let him do so at once. The persons who go about denouncing such invaluable gifts to the human race are the heirs of those ancient wiseacres who laughed at Sir William Harvey when he said that the blood flowed through the veins, and hooted at Jenner when he proposed to vaccinate all England, and called Klemke a lunatic when he maintained that tuberculosis was infectious.

That antitoxin, employed in time, will cure diphtheria is a fact as easily demonstrable as the fact that the sun rises every morning. And the fact that nothing else in the world—no medicine, throat mopping or surgical operation—will cure it, is demonstrable, too. Medicines and moppings have their usefulness as aids, but it is the antitoxin—or, when the antitoxin is not used, long-suffering nature—that wins the battle.

It is evident, however, that the antitoxin, while it neutralizes the poisons secreted by the bacilli, does not directly kill the bacilli themselves. The business of getting rid of them falls upon the white blood corpuscles, and the great majority of them are soon gobbled up, but not a few remain. These, unless something is done to kill them, are apt to infect other persons. Active germs have been found in the throats of recovered diphtheria patients three months after the disease itself apparently disappeared, and there is one remarkable case on record, where they remained alive for twenty-two months. They also live in the air, in water, and elsewhere.

In consequence, it is highly important that children who are convalescent be kept away from other children. They should be isolated for at least a month, and it is unwise to send them to school for several weeks longer. The business of stamping out the stray bacilli which may happen to infect the sick-room should be entrusted to some one who knows how to do it. The common device of hanging up cloths saturated with carbolic acid is utterly useless. In many cities the municipal health department takes charge of all disinfections.

When this is the case, it is very unwise for mothers to offer opposition. The health department experts know what they are about, and their work may very easily prevent other cases in the same house or epidemics in the neighborhood. One little life saved is worth all the bother and disorder that these men, with their enmity to wall-papers, cause in a household.

During the progress of a case of diphtheria, the rooms occupied by the patient—and it is best to have two bedrooms, that there may be frequent changes—should be isolated absolutely from the rest of the house, and it is advisable, whenever possible, to send all the other children of the house away and withdraw them from school until all possibility that they, too, are infected has been eliminated.

It is best, whenever possible, to call in a graduate nurse, but too often the fear-stricken mother must herself assume the office of bedside attendant. To those confronted by this difficult duty, I would suggest the importance of submitting to a preventive injection of antitoxin. Small doses for this purpose are especially prepared by the various manufacturers. The inoculation causes little discomfort and no illness, but it is a certain preventive. Most adults are immune to diphtheria, but the importance of keeping the nurse in good health throughout the period of nursing is obvious, and so it is well to take no chances.

You should have the doctor give you a prescription for a mouth gargle and use it every hour. In addition you should wash your hands at frequent intervals with antiseptic soap. All spoons, glasses and other vessels should be cleansed with a three per cent solution of carbolic acid. Toys, cushions, carpets, pictures and furniture—in fact, everything movable—should be taken from the sick-room. Its furnishings should be limited entirely to the bed, a table and a chair for the nurse. The floor and walls should be sponged once a day with a one-tenth of one per cent solution of bichloride of mercury. The bedclothes and garments of both patient and nurse should be boiled, and all sick-room débris should be burned. The eyes, nose and mouth of the patient should be frequently swabbed with moist absorbent cotton, and the cotton should then be burned.

Not a solitary person besides the nurse and the doctor should be permitted to enter the sick-room under any circumstances. As I have said, most adults are immune to diphtheria, but it is perfectly possible for them to carry away the germs and infect children. I recently encountered in my own practice the case of a drawing teacher who infected at least a score of children without being ill herself. The germs of the disease were in her throat.

The nursing of a case of diphtheria requires eternal watchfulness and care. Even when the disease is making favorable progress, there is danger of sudden heart failure and collapse, and the management of such emergencies is beyond the skill of the mother. If your little patient seems to be fainting, and the pulse grows weak, send for the nearest doctor at once. In any case the convalescent is always very much exhausted, and should be kept in bed a good while. The diet should be rigidly prescribed by the physician. It is exceedingly dangerous to add a coveted dish to it—no matter how harmless that dish may seem—without his express permission.

Methods of preventing diphtheria will present themselves to the intelligent mother. The notion that every child is doomed to suffer from the disease at some time during its first decade (and to suffer attacks of a long string of other infantile epidemics, likewise) is a dangerous and stupid error. There is no reason whatever why any child need have diphtheria, scarlet fever or measles, just as there is no reason why it need have smallpox, lockjaw or hydrophobia. All of these infections are preventable.

In a great many cases kissing spreads diphtheria—particularly from adults, in whose mouths the germs may be impotent, to children. Therefore, the custom of permitting small children to be fondled and kissed by every sentimental woman relative and visitor should be under the ban. Again, it is well to break children of the habit of putting things into their mouths. It is easy to do this, and the precaution may save lives. Rubber pacifiers, the toys used to divert children in photograph galleries, and other things of that sort frequently swarm with the bacilli.

As I have tried to show, success in battling with diphtheria depends almost entirely upon promptness. A delay in sending for the doctor is often fatal. Whenever a child's throat is sore, and a membrane obstructs the air passages, it is safe to conclude that there is some diphtheritic infection. Even a mild redness, without membrane, or pain, may indicate the presence of the disease. Such a mild case may pursue an uneventful and unalarming course—and then suddenly end in heart failure. It is best, at all times, to put no trust in home remedies for the treatment of sore throats. Only a physician is capable of differentiating between diphtheria and less dangerous infections.

The so-called "pseudo-diphtheria" of the old-school family doctors is not diphtheria at all, but a milder tonsil infection due to the presence of organisms called the *streptococcus* and *staphylococcus*. But the existence of such an infection shows that the little patient's throat membranes afford good soil for germs, and so it should be guarded against diphtheria with unusual vigilance. Bad teeth, mouth sores, enlarged tonsils, catarrhal inflammations and other abnormalities in the respiratory tract also predispose to the disease. Susceptibility is increased, again, by measles and scarlet fever. In the majority of cases, the germs first find a lodgment in the tonsils. Therefore, it is a wise precaution to have enlarged and sensitive tonsils removed in early infancy.

When a child has been exposed to infection, and the fact is known, an immunizing injection of antitoxin should be made at once. If this is done in time, the disease is effectually headed off. As I have said, the antitoxin is harmless, and cannot possibly injure a healthy child. The prejudice against it (and traces of this prejudice are to be encountered among ignorant, old-fashioned doctors as well as among silly mothers) is doubtless due to the fact that it has been in use but a short while. Not until 1894 was its value demonstrated, and only since 1895 has it been in general use. In these few years, I should say, it has saved the lives of at least three hundred thousand children.

Commentary

Chapter 11: If Your Baby Had Diphtheria

"If Your Baby Had Diphtheria" is a crisp and informative discourse on the leading cause of childhood mortality in the early 20th century. The essay opens with a realistic portrayal of the fear, mystery, and terror that shrouded the disease, and explains the use of diphtheria antitoxin, a widely employed therapeutic agent before the advent of the diphtheria vaccine, and the importance of quarantine or isolating the patient with diphtheria in order to halt the spread of the epidemic.

Diphtheria is an infectious disease in which a microbe, *Corynebacterium diphtheriae,* attacks the mucus membranes of the throat and airway. A toxin secreted by the organism leads to an intense inflammatory response, and a thick tenacious pseudomembrane forms over the back of the throat. Thus the initial complaint of a child stricken with diphtheria is that of an extremely sore throat. Without methods of culturing the diphtheria bacillus, the early diagnosis was difficult and often confused with pseudo-diphtheria, a less dangerous inflammation of the throat and airway usually caused by a streptococcal infection. In addition to causing a sore throat, high fever, and exhaustion, the pseudomembrane of diphtheria often became thick enough to obstruct the flow of air; the all-too-common result of such an infection was the child's suffocation, usually in the presence of helpless and terrified parents. Techniques of airway management such as intubation, which consists of inserting a tube through the pseudomembrane into the trachea; and tracheotomy, incising the tracheal cartilage below the blockage and inserting an artificial airway through the incision, were developed to deal with this leading cause of death in diphtheria epidemics.[1] Another equally feared complication of diphtheria was that survivors of the initial phase of the disease (the inflammation of the throat and upper respiratory tract) were susceptible to the secondary effects of diphtheria toxin once it began circulating in the bloodstream. For many patients such toxic effects caused heart failure, paralysis, and death anywhere from 2 to 6 weeks after diphtheria's initial attack.

Mencken and Hirshberg emphasize the speedy administration of diphtheria antitoxin to the child suspected of having the disease. As they note, antitoxin is an immune factor that blocks the deleterious, systemic effects of diphtheria toxin. It was developed in 1890 by the German scientist Emil von Behring, whose research not only led to a treatment for the disease but also showed that specific immune factors are found in the liquid portion of the blood or serum. Behring was awarded the first Nobel prize in Medicine and Physiology for this work in 1901.[2]

Further experimentation was required, however, to make diphtheria antitoxin a safe and effective therapeutic measure. In 1893 Pierre Roux, a colleague of Pasteur, found that the horse was the best source of antitoxin, as vividly described in this chapter. Paul Ehrlich, the German immunologist who later discovered salvarsan 606 (the "magic bullet") for syphilis, spent the years 1893 and 1894 standardizing the strength of diphtheria antitoxin produced by different laboratories.[3] This work guaranteed that a dose produced by one laboratory would be equal in strength to a dose produced by another laboratory, an extremely important accomplishment at a time when many drugs or medications were produced by individual sources instead of by mass production. Other scientists devoted years of study and research to answering questions as to how much diphtheria antitoxin to administer, when and how to administer it, and other pertinent information. All of this crucial work resulted in the development of a therapeutic agent that lowered the mortality of diphtheria by at least 90%, justifying Mencken's proclamation:

> No other single medical discovery of recent years has better proved its value to the human race, or better justified the bold experimentation—the ruthless slaughter of rabbits and guinea pigs—the patient toil with culture and microscope—of medical science.

Always a supporter of responsible and scientific research, Mencken was later to define the antivivisectionist as "one who gags at a guinea pig and swallows a baby."[4] The treatment today for someone unfortunate enough to contract diphtheria is still the same as that described in "If Your Baby Had Diphtheria."

The diphtheria toxoid vaccine was not developed until 1923 by Gaston Ramon of the Pasteur Institute. The vaccine is produced by a process that modifies the diphtheria toxin with heat and formalin, rendering the toxin harmless to the recipient (hence, the name toxoid) but still capable of producing immunity. Ramon's toxoid vaccine was tested on Baltimore City school children in an extensive field trial in 1936 by researchers at the Johns Hopkins School of Hygiene and Public Health. The results, of course, were an outstanding success that is still enjoyed today. Currently diphtheria is extremely rare in North America. For example, in 1980 fewer than 0.01 cases per 100,000 people were reported compared to 220 cases per 100,000 people in 1919; 12,000 people, mostly children, died from the disease or its complications in 1919 compared to 1 death in 1982.[6] Any recent cases of diphtheria in the U.S. are exclusively due to failure to vaccinate against the disease.[7,8] The ordeal and terror of diphtheria, once a commonplace and harsh reality of childhood, can now be completely and safely avoided with proper immunization.

QUESTIONS FOR THE MOTHER ABOUT CHAPTER 11

1. What is the one thing that has reduced the death-rate from diphtheria so marvelously in the last ten years?
1910 Diphtheria antitoxin.

2. How soon should the antitoxin be administered?

1910 As soon as diphtheria is suspected to be present.

3. How can this be proved?

1910 A "culture" should be taken of the patient's throat.

4. How is this culture taken?

1910 The doctor scrapes the patient's throat and has the mucous examined at once by a bacteriologist to see if the diphtheria germ is present.

5. How can a mother protect the family from taking diphtheria from the patient before she is sure it is diphtheria?

1910 She should call a doctor for tonsillitis or a bad sore throat and should isolate a child suffering from a cold or sore throat.

6. How can she prevent the disease from attacking those who have been exposed to it?

1910 She should at once notify the Board of Health. Either a Board of Health doctor or her private physician will make a mild injection of antitoxin for each person exposed. If the mother takes care of the child she should have such an injection also, as her health is all-important at this crisis.

7. What can we do to prevent diphtheria?

1910 Brush the teeth thoroughly after each meal; use a mouth wash; have adenoid growths or enlarged tonsils removed; take care not to infect other people if we have a cold or sore throat. Take care not to let other people infect us if they have a cold or sore throat. Never kiss one another on the mouth.

8. How can we prevent diphtheria epidemics at school?

1910 Diphtheria germs are present in the mouths of many healthy persons. These persons are called "germ carriers." A "culture" should be taken of every child's throat before it enters school in the fall. In this way the "germ carriers" can be weeded out.

REFERENCES

1. Alberti PW. Tracheotomy vs. intubation. A 19th century controversy. *Annals of Otology, Rhinology, and Laryngology* 93:333–337, 1984.

2. Behring EA. Uber des zustandekommen der diphtherie-immunitat und der tetanus-immunitat bei thieren. *Dtsh. Med. Wochenschr.* 16:113–114, 1980. A superb review of the history of diphtheria can be found by Dr. Peter C. English. (Diphtheria and theories of infectious disease: Centennial appreciation of the critical role of diphtheria in the history of medicine. *Pediatrics* 76:1–9, 1985.)

3. Rosen G. Acute communicable diseases. *In* Bett WR (ed.). *The History and Conquest of Common Diseases.* Norman, Oklahoma: University of Oklahoma Press, 1954, pp. 6–26.

4. Mencken HL. This and that. *A Mencken Chrestomathy.* New York: Alfred A. Knopf, Inc., 1949, p. 626.

5. Frost WH. Diphtheria in Baltimore: a comparative study of morbidity, carrier prevalence, and antitoxic immunity in 1921–1924 and 1933–36. *In* Maxcy KF (ed.). *Papers of Wade Hampton Frost. M.D. A Contribution to Epidemiological Method.* New York: Commonwealth Fund, 1941.

6. Dixon JMS. Diphtheria in North America. *Journal of Hygiene* 93:419–432, 1984.

7. Centers for Disease Control. Fatal Diphtheria—Wisconsin. *Morbidity and Mortality Weekly Report* 31:553–555, 1982.

8. Centers for Disease Control. *Immunization Against Disease, 1980.*

12
If Your Baby Had Scarlet Fever

Now that smallpox, thanks to compulsory vaccination, has become a rarity in civilized communities, scarlet fever steps forward as the worst of the eruptive diseases of childhood.

It is a malady of enormous antiquity. Thucydides, writing nearly five hundred years before the beginning of our era, called it a heritage from the remote past. It has scourged the white races in all ages and all countries, and the physicians of all schools have leveled their heaviest artillery upon it. Yet it remains a puzzle unsolved and an enemy unconquered even to-day. We are in doubt as to its cause, and there is as yet no drug or antitoxin that will cure it.

But despite all this, the death-rate from scarlet fever is steadily declining, and we may expect it to decline more and more as the years go by. The reason for this, I take it, lies in the fact that the modern doctor is a great deal more sparing with pills and powders than his predecessor, and a great deal more lavish with water, air and antiseptics. In the old days it was customary to dose scarlet fever patients with all sorts of violent remedies, in staggering quantities, and, as a result, many of them died. Today medicines are but minor auxiliaries in the sick-room, and both doctor and nurse devote their main energies to preventing a spread of the infection.

Though the exact cause of scarlet fever is still far from certain, there is no doubt whatever that it will be determined with absolute accuracy within a few years. A large number of competent observers, in truth, have already come to the conclusion that the causative agent must be a minute parasite closely related to that which produces malaria. The organisms of diphtheria, tuberculosis and most other common maladies belong to the vegetable kingdom, like the germs of the yeast, but this so-called scarlet fever organism is a true animal. It is at the very bottom of the scale of brute creation, and is almost as far below the caterpillar as the latter is below the highest grade of man-like ape.

An attack of scarlet fever may begin a day or so after the patient has been exposed to contagion, and then again there may be an incubation period of a week or even more. Several years ago, in the course of my practice, I one day visited a family in which there were four bad cases. Next day I left the city and remained away for a full week. On the day of my return I fell ill with the disease, and a very severe attack was immediately in progress. In this case the incubation period seems to have been no less than eight days.

Scarlet fever usually begins with chills, rising fever, headache, loss of appetite and pains in the limbs, and sometimes, particularly in very young children, with convulsions. A sore throat and painful tonsils next afflict the patient, and at the end of a day or so the characteristic red rash appears. This commonly begins around the neck and over the chest, and at the start consists of tiny scarlet blotches the size of pinheads. The blotches soon run together and the whole surface of the body becomes a brilliant red. The membranes of the mouth are affected in much the same way, and the tongue becomes swollen and takes on the so-called "raspberry" appearance.

Despite the almost universal notion, there is no crisis in scarlet fever. A crisis, in medicine, means a sudden change in or termination of symptoms. In scarlet fever the fever does not cease suddenly, but slowly. This is called a termination by lysis, which is the very reverse of crisis. When the fever goes down—usually about the fifth day—the scarlet rash begins to disappear and the skin of the patient begins to peel off. Sometimes it comes off in large patches, and the skin of nearly a whole hand may separate in a single piece.

When this peeling has fairly begun, the malady itself may be said to have practically run its course, but there yet remains a grave danger from serious complications. The worst of these are Bright's disease, several varieties of heart disease and inflammation of the inner ear. Bright's disease, as every one knows, may readily lead to long invalidism and death, and inflammation of the inner ear only too often produces meningitis, abscesses on the brain, or permanent deafness. The belief that scarlet fever tends to leave some nasty souvenir of its visit is far from a mere superstition. It has an unpleasant habit, too, of paving the way for other acute diseases, such as pneumonia, bronchitis and even diphtheria.

All this makes it apparent that a case of scarlet fever needs very careful nursing. Whenever it is possible a trained nurse should be engaged, and in any event the doctor's orders should be obeyed with scrupulous exactness. Nothing could be more foolish than the common custom of seeking advice in such emergencies from grandmothers, neighbors who have "pulled their own children through" and other well-meaning but blundering "experts" of that species. Good nursing means not only intelligent care of the patient, and a capacity for quickly and accurately recognizing threatening complications, but also intelligent efforts to prevent a spread of the infection. Scarlet fever is one of the most contagious of known maladies, and in achieving an effective quarantine of his patient the cautious physician often takes measures which, to the layman, may seem almost ridiculously elaborate.

When one of your children develops the disease, put it to bed in a large and airy room, preferably on the top floor of the house, and prepare another room nearby, into which the child may be taken when the sick-room proper is being aired and cleaned. Take all unnecessary furnishings out of both rooms. Under this heading come carpets, rugs, pictures, draperies and ornaments. In the sick-room a bed for the patient and a chair and table for the nurse are about all that may be called needful. A plain clothes-rack will suffice for holding the necessary changes of bed-clothes.

If it is at all possible, send the other children of the household to some relative's home and keep them away from school for a week. If they are apparently well at the end of that time, it will be safe to let them go back to school. If sending them away is out of the question and they must remain in the house, keep them away from all other children until the patient up-stairs is well. They may take the disease at any time, even in the face of careful precautions, and you certainly would be greatly grieved to see them carry it to their fellow pupils and playmates.

If you are able to engage a trained nurse—or, better still, two of them—the problem of nursing is much simplified, for the nurses will carry out the doctor's orders intelligently and faithfully, and in their comings and goings they will see to it that they do not carry the infection. Your own visits to the sick-room should be as far apart as your anxiety will permit you to make them, you should stay but a short while, and avoid handling the patient. Before you enter the room put on a long duster or rain coat that completely covers your ordinary clothes. Place a close-fitting hood, such as housemaids wear when dusting, over your hair. These garments should be kept at the sick-room door. When you leave, wash your hands thoroughly, putting a few drops of carbolic acid into the water. After that, spend half an hour in the open air and sunlight.

If you decide to nurse your child yourself, you must resign yourself to an entire separation from the other children in the house for a period of at least six weeks. Your bedroom should be next to or very near that of the patient, of course, but I cannot advise your sleeping in the sick-chamber itself. Besides increasing the chances of infection, this practice results in unduly vitiating the air of the room. The oxygen that you consume is needed by the child, for in a sick-room the supply of oxygen is never too ample.

With proper treatment, the patient should be quiet enough to give you a reasonable amount of rest, but you must school yourself to awaken easily in order that you may look after its nocturnal wants. It is highly important that you go out every day for an hour or so for fresh air and exercise, and during this time some one else must be on guard. This assistant nurse, during her stay in the sick-room, should wear the long coat and the dust-cap I have already described. You, yourself, on leaving the sick-room, should make a complete change of clothes, and wash your face and hands thoroughly. The clothes you wear outside should be kept in an ante-room.

These precautions may seem unduly elaborate, but in view of the extraordinary infectiousness of scarlet fever, they are not. In my own practice I wear a skull-cap and long rain coat whenever I enter the room of a patient ill with the disease. In addition, I cover my mustache and beard with strips of sterile cotton, and see to the surgical cleanliness of my hands—and this is far greater than ordinary soap-and-water cleanliness—when I depart.

In the sick-room, for general antiseptic purposes, you should keep a wooden (not a metal) bucket filled with a one-tenth percent solution of corrosive sublimate. The drug stores sell this powerful germicide in convenient tablet form. Use one tablet for every pint of water. All towels, sheets and other cloths used in the sick-room should be soaked in this solution for an hour before they are placed in the family laundry basket. It should be used, too, instead of plain water, for moistening all cloths employed in wiping the floor and furniture.

You know, of course, that corrosive sublimate is a most violent poison, but this fact need not worry you, for a weak solution, such as I have recommended, can do little damage. After it wets your hands, wash them with soap and water. It may make the skin a bit dark and rough, but this will wear off very quickly. In mopping the floor, see that the cloth is moist, and not soaking wet. The sick-room must never be dusty (this bans all sweeping), but neither should it be steamy and damp.

The doctor will give you detailed instructions as to the care of the patient. The little sufferer will probably be greatly annoyed by the discharges from its nose, throat and ears, and these must constantly be looked to. Instead of a handkerchief or napkin for keeping it clean, use small bits of the absorbent cotton sold by every druggist. This cotton is cheap, it has been sterilized, and its application is not irritating. Every piece should be burned immediately after it has been used.

It will be a great aid to the doctor if you can give him an accurate report upon the varying temperature of the patient. To the layman, taking a temperature may appear difficult, but it is really a very simple matter. A clinical thermometer costs less than a dollar, and the doctor will show you how to read it. If the patient is afraid to hold it under the tongue, place it in the rectum. The normal temperature of a human being is 98.6 degrees Fahrenheit. In scarlet fever it may rise to 103 or even 105 degrees. Whenever it begins to grow high, the doctor should be informed at once.

After the fever goes down and the child's skin begins to shed, it will suffer greatly from itching. This can be relieved by rubbing the body very gently with carbolated Vaseline. During this stage the child should be bathed often in cold lime-water or in water which contains a small amount of ordinary baking-soda. Hot baths are to be avoided, but the water may be warmed enough, as the phrase goes, "to take the chill off." Do not attempt to help nature by pulling off the pieces of loose skin. They will drop off themselves just as soon as the new skin beneath them is hard enough to be exposed.

The ancient belief that a sick-room may be disinfected by hanging up cloths saturated with weak carbolic acid or some other antiseptic is without a basis in fact. An antiseptic, to kill a germ, must be brought into actual contact with it.

That is why all towels and sheets must be not merely dampened by, but actually soaked in, the corrosive sublimate. If you managed to get enough carbolic acid into the air to kill the germs, you would kill the human occupants, too.

Scarlet fever is most contagious from the third to the seventh day, but its contagiousness does not disappear entirely for a long while after that. Until the shedding of the skin and the discharge from the ears have quite ceased, no person save the doctor and the nurses should be permitted to approach the patient, and in any case the period of quarantine should be at least six weeks.

If you have had scarlet fever in childhood you need not fear for your own health, but, even if you haven't, your chances of taking it are small. It is, in fact, rare among adults, but all the same it is well to adopt precautions.

After the patient has recovered, the sick-room should be thoroughly cleansed; and this means cleansed in the surgical, and not in the common, sense. In large cities the work is best entrusted to the health department. When such experts are not available, the floor, walls and ceilings should be mopped again and again with the corrosive sublimate solution, and the windows should be thrown wide open. It is always best to have the wall-paper scraped off.

There is no reason to fear the worst when the doctor's verdict is scarlet fever. In all maladies, you should remember that the death-rate is kept up by the enormous number of deaths among the children of the very poor.

Commentary

Chapter 12: If Your Baby Had Scarlet Fever

The words **SCARLET FEVER** emphatically posted in red letters upon the door of a house in 1910 were enough to instill fear in the strongest of men. Among parents of small children, the words could easily evoke hand-wringing terror. Not unlike AIDS during the early 1980s, scarlet fever was a poorly understood disease with many manifestations, an unclear pattern of transmission, no clear cause, and no cure.

Confusing in its presentation, scarlet fever usually appears in the classic form described by Mencken and Hirshberg. It begins with a sore throat and high fever followed by a diffuse, bright red, "sandpapery" or "goose-bump"-like rash; the skin eventually peels a few days after the rash appeared. In other children, however, scarlet fever might present only as a sore throat with headache, malaise, and fever but without skin eruption, yet close family members subsequently infected could develop the full-blown syndrome. Although the majority of children infected with scarlet fever recovered uneventfully, a significant number would go on to develop a condition then known as "rheumatism" or acute rheumatic fever; this condition is heralded by a migratory arthritis, an inflammation of the heart and its lining that can progress to severe damage of the cardiac valves (endocarditis), and purposeless, uncontrollable, repetitive movements of the body (chorea). Other scarlet fever victims developed a generalized swelling from fluid retention and a slow, progressive form of kidney failure beginning with bloody urine and increased excretion of protein in the urine due to faulty filtering by the kidneys. This chronic kidney failure was then termed Bright's disease, named for the British physician Sir Richard Bright (1789–1858) who described it in 1827; it is presently referred to as poststreptococcal glomerulonephritis.

Although descriptions of scarlet fever date back to medieval times, one of the first accurate descriptions of the disease and its protean manifestations was provided by the famed British physician Thomas Sydenham (1624–1689) when he differentiated the disease from the similarly presenting measles. Sydenham, who referred to scarlet fever as *Febris scarlatina,* based his observations on a London epidemic in 1675.[1] The recognition and diagnosis of scarlet fever were further advanced by the French clinician Armand Trousseau who, in 1870, noted the long-term complications of the disease, namely rheumatic fever and kidney failure.[2] Yet it was precisely the multifaceted and changing manifestations of scarlet fever that caused it to be confused by physicians with measles, diphtheria, and other acute infections. One explanation for this confusion might be that physicians trained in "humoralism" were easily bewildered by different diseases that presented with similar symptoms; a throat made sore by scarlet fever was difficult to distinguish from the sore throat of diphtheria, especially if one had never seen the characteristic grayish-green pseudomembrane brought on by diphtheria. Likewise, to a physician lacking clinical experience, the red, goose-bumpy rash of scarlet fever might be confused with the more confluent, unraised rash of measles. Such examples indicate just how important knowing the cause of an illness is in making a diagnosis. If the throat culture of an ill child complaining of a sore throat showed diphtheria as opposed to streptococcus, the physician could modify his plan of treatment to fit that disease's exact symptoms and expect or hope to prevent its complications. And while medicine had much to learn in 1910 about managing acute infectious diseases, the advent of the germ theory—the elucidation of specific microbes as the cause of specific diseases, and their subsequent treatment—made the physician's job a great deal more satisfying, not to mention rational and scientific.

The versatile manifestations of scarlet fever, however, were not the only confusing factors in the delineation of the disease. Physicians were also mystified by the cause and wide variance in the incidence and virulence of scarlet fever epidemics. For example, 17th century physicians were puzzled by the fact that poor children living in the slums of London suffered a far more severe form of scarlet fever and had a higher susceptibility to the disease's more malignant complications than their wealthy, well-bred cohorts. Similarly, doctors in the United States during the 1800s could not explain why their patients with scarlet fever seemed to have a much milder form of the disease and a lower incidence of death compared with victims in previously recorded epidemics. Such fluctuations in the severity of scarlet fever epidemics over the years were obviously far more complicated than the overuse of "pills and powders" and lack of "water, air, and antiseptics" as proposed by Mencken.

The concerted and systematic study of the social pattern of microbes and their interactions with man has provided plausible explanations for the changing nature of epidemics of scarlet fever. Virulence, the infectious organism's ability to cause disease, for example, depends upon a great many factors such as the microbe's ability to be transmitted from one person to another, its ability to resist the host's defense or immune system, the properties that the microbe may have to invade the host and multiply within it, and whether or not that microbe can generate and secrete poisonous toxins that cause harm to that host.[3] The amount of infectious matter, or inoculum, the host encounters can play a role in whether or not one contracts an infectious disease. For example, if 100 susceptible children were exposed to the nasopharyngeal secretions of one child with chickenpox, 95 would contract the disease. Chickenpox, therefore, is an extremely contagious disease and only a small inoculum is necessary to cause it. The acquired immunodeficiency syndrome (AIDS), on the other hand, is almost exclusively transmitted by sexual contact or by the exchange of blood, such as in the sharing of needles and comingling of blood by intravenous drug abusers or in receiving a blood or blood product transfusion infected with the human immunodeficiency virus (HIV). A large inoculum of HIV is probably necessary to cause AIDS. One of the reasons scarlet fever is so contagious is because only a small inoculum of the hearty organism, *Streptococcus pyogenes,* needs to be inhaled to cause the disease.

Finally, the health status of the particular host at hand plays an important role in the severity of illness. Weak, ill, malnourished, and extremely young hosts are more susceptible to infectious diseases than healthy ones, as noted by the doctors observing the 1675 epidemic of scarlet fever in London.

During the 19th century scientists agreed that scarlet fever was a communicable disease, but there was great debate as to which microbe was responsible. The family of bacteria called Streptococcus had long been implicated in scarlet fever, but because the family had not yet been divided into its many classes, types, and strains, it was not yet possible to satisfy all of Koch's postulates of disease with the ubiquitous streptococci. Technical bacteriological tests needed to be developed in order to separate pathogenic (or disease-producing) from nonpathogenic strains of streptococcus. For example, some strains of streptococci were noted to break up or lyse red blood cells in culture, whereas others did not. These "hemolytic" strains of streptococci were thought to be causally related to scarlet fever, but, again, definitive proof in the eyes of the bacteriologist—the strict fulfillment of Koch's postulates—was lacking. Other scientists asserted that streptococci, hemolytic or nonhemolytic, were not the causative organisms of scarlet fever at all. The noted Harvard pathologist F.B. Mallory, among others, was convinced that scarlet fever was due to an infection caused by a protozoon (a one-celled organism of a higher order of evolution when compared to bacteria) based upon a study of four patients with scarlet fever in 1904. Mallory insisted that streptococci were found in patients with scarlet fever only as a secondary infection. Hirshberg, who kept up to date on medical progress (or, at least, had the diligence to look up scarlet fever in the latest edition of Osler's *System of Medicine*),[5] included this erroneous opinion in the materials he gathered for Mencken on scarlet fever.

The search for the causative microbe of scarlet fever was long and arduous, lasting far longer than similar searches in diseases such as diphtheria, whooping cough, and tuberculosis. It was not until 1923, 13 years after publication of *What You Ought to Know About Your Baby*, that a husband and wife team, George and Gladys Dick, proved that a species of the Streptococcus family, *Streptococcus pyogenes*, caused scarlet fever.[6] An erythrogenic (red-producing) toxin secreted by this microbe is responsible not only for the transient red rash of scarlet fever but also for the more deadly complications such as the inflammation of the heart and kidneys. Further research by Rebecca Lancefield identified *Streptococcus pyogenes* as part of a group of microbes called Group A hemolytic streptococci, all of which produce disease in humans.[7] This discovery explained why some children infected with streptococci developed only a sore throat, whereas others developed scarlet fever. In fact, group A hemolytic streptococci continue to be an unhappy reality of childhood and are responsible for a number of diseases, including skin infections, ear infections, sore throats, and pneumonia. Fortunately all are easily treated with antibiotics such as the penicillin-based drugs, loving care, and a healthy dose of television. The judicious use of antibiotics has made the long-term, deadly complications of scarlet fever a rare occurrence.

This chapter points out that the only therapy for scarlet fever in 1909 was good nursing care and stresses the importance of a trained (or "graduate") nurse following the orders of a physician. The theme of the good nurse was to recur in Mencken's book *In Defense of Women:*

> ...she [a woman] is usually a success as a sick nurse, for that profession requires ingenuity, quick comprehension, courage in the face of novel and disconcerting situations, and above all, a capacity for a penetrating and dominating character.[8]

QUESTIONS FOR THE MOTHER ABOUT CHAPTER 12

1. What is the one thought you should have in your mind where there is scarlet fever?

1910 The danger of one case of scarlet fever in a town to the rest of the community.

2. Why?

1910 Because scarlet fever is one of the most contagious of diseases. Because it is very dangerous and leads to other serious diseases.

3. What is necessary to protect a community against scarlet fever?

1910 That every case, as soon as it is discovered, should be reported to the health department.

4. What will the health department do?

1910 It will send a doctor to examine the child. It will give the mother information about preventing the spread of the disease to the other children in her family or in the town. It will place a sign "scarlet fever" on the door to warn people. It will fumigate the home.

5. What should a mother do if the health department does not take such care of a scarlet fever case?

1910 She should send at once for her doctor and ask him how to care for the child and how to disinfect. She should place a large red letter sign SCARLET FEVER on her door to protect her neighbors. She should keep all the persons who have been exposed to scarlet fever away from other persons, and the children away from school or play on the street until the time in which they might come down with the disease is passed.

6. What are the precautions to be taken to prevent infection from scarlet fever?

1910 All sheets, nightgowns, towels, etc., used by the patient and nurse should be soaked twenty-four hours in a solution of carbolic acid before taken from the sick-room, then thoroughly boiled.

Every dish used in the sick-room should be washed in carbolic acid solution before taken from the room.

Every book, toy or article that cannot be boiled should be burned. A child has caught scarlet fever from a book that had been in the room when her brother had scarlet fever two years before.

No letter written by the patient should be permitted to leave the room. Allowing an infected letter to go through the mails, carrying a child with a contagious disease through the street car or trains is a crime to one's fellowmen that should be punishable by law. If it is necessary to take a child in a hack to the hospital or home, the hack should be fumigated and disinfected before being entered by another person.

7. How long is there danger of infection from a scarlet fever case?

1910 Until every bit of the old skin—skin that peels off—comes off the body *naturally*.

8. What should be done when the patient recovers?

1910 It should be bathed and its hair washed in disinfectant before leaving the room. Place a clean wrapper at the door and have clean clothes for it in another room where it may get dressed. Then burn a formaldehyde candle in the room, wash the floors and the woodwork and the walls with a solution of corrosive sublimate. Then the wall paper should be torn off the wall and the room should be repapered.

How much cheaper is this than another case of scarlet fever, perhaps resulting in death.

REFERENCES

1. Sydenham T. *Opera omnia*. London: Impensis Societatis Sydenhamianae, 1844, pp. 243–244.
2. Trousseau A. Scarlatina. Reprinted in *Reviews of Infectious Diseases* 1:1016–1026, 1979. Originally appeared in *Lectures on Clinical Medicine*. Philadelphia: Lindsay and Blakiston, 1869.
3. Rosen G. Acute communicable diseases. In Bett WR. *The History and Conquest of Common Diseases*. Norman, Oklahoma: University of Oklahoma Press, 1954, pp. 26–38.
4. Mallory FB. Scarlet fever: protozoon-like bodies found in four cases. *Journal of Medical Research* 5:483–492, 1904.
5. McCollom JH. Scarlet fever In Osler W, McCrae T (eds.). *Osler's System of Medicine*, Vol. 2. Oxford: Oxford University Press, 1907, p. 341.
6. Dick GF, Dick GH. The etiology of scarlet fever. *Journal of the American Medical Association*. 82:301–302, 1924.
7. Lancefield RC. *Journal of Experimental Medicine*; 47:91–103, 481–491, 1928.
8. Mencken HL. *In Defense of Women*. New York: Time Books, 1963.

13
Whooping Cough: It Kills More Children Than Scarlet Fever and Diphtheria Together

Whooping cough is one of the most contagious of all maladies of childhood, and, in very young children, one of the most dangerous. Personal contact is not necessary in order to transfer the infection from one child to another. Children may take it by merely entering a house in which there is a patient, and some observers assert that it may even be transmitted from child to child on the street. After the third year it is not often fatal, but among very small children it plays havoc. During the whole of the first year indeed, it shows a death rate of at least 25 percent. This proves how important it is to guard babies against contagion. The notion that whooping cough is a mild disease, which every child would better acquire early, for its subsequent good, is a costly fallacy.

We are yet somewhat in the dark as to the cause of whooping cough, but there is very good reason to hold that it is produced by a small organism allied to the germs of the other infectious diseases. This organism, it is possible, enters through the mouth or nose and takes up its home in the larynx, where it at once proceeds to irritate and destroy the mucous membrane, and to send forth poisons into all parts of the body. The first result is an accumulation of cellular debris and mucous in the larynx, and the second is a serious interference with the normal working of the bodily machinery, particularly that part of it which makes up the nervous system.

The accumulation in the larynx, it seems likely, is the direct cause of the suffocating cough, though certain observers believe that the principal seat of trouble is elsewhere. Whatever the precise mechanism, it is plain that the effort in the cough is directed toward ridding the larynx of its obstruction, and that the expulsion of this obstruction, which comes up in the form of a sticky mass, is followed by a cessation of the paroxysm.

Whooping cough starts like a common cold, and sometimes it runs so mild a course that it is scarcely recognizable. But ordinarily, its peculiar characteristics begin to appear after a few days. One of these is the tendency of the cough to grow worse at night, and another is its tendency to become convulsive and racking. The child gasps for breath after each attack and seems to be much exhausted.

In a week or ten days the familiar whoop sets all doubts at rest. Anyone who has ever heard this whoop will never forget it. It is caused by the labored in-breathing of air through the narrowed glottis, and well exhibits the distress of the patient. The cough itself is violent in the extreme. The child, as if suffocating, grasps at nearby objects, its face grows red, the veins of its neck swell, the tongue protrudes and the muscles of the whole upper part of the body are strained. After each effort to clear the air passages there comes the whoop. Finally, there is a spasm of extra violence, the mass of mucous is expelled, and the child sinks back exhausted.

It is common for vomiting to follow, and in some cases this vomiting is so severe that it becomes one of the most distressing symptoms. At times, indeed, the patient seems unable to retain any food in the stomach. In such cases, of course, the exhaustion becomes progressively more severe, and the physician finds the nutrition of the patient a serious problem.

The number of coughing spells in the twenty-four hours varies greatly, and is modified somewhat by the care exercised in nursing. A sudden draught will often bring on a severe paroxysm, as will a drink of cold water. Children are also apt to start coughing on hearing some one else cough, and any other noise or shock may have the same effect. The paroxysms are always more frequent at night, and between the severe ones there may be a large number of lesser ones.

Very little can be done to shorten or mitigate the paroxysm, once it starts. If the child is old enough to stand alone, it is best, perhaps, not to touch it. If it is in arms, it should be held gently, but firmly. Inhalations are often of value, but they can be used to better advantage between the paroxysms rather than during their progress. Often the mucous coughed up is bloody, and there may be bleeding from the nose or throat. Unless this is very profuse it need cause no alarm.

The whooping stage continues for from three weeks to two months, after which the cough grows milder, the vomiting ceases and the child begins to regain strength. Even when there are no complications, whooping cough is a very exhausting malady, and so it is necessary to observe the child closely during convalescence. It should get plenty of fresh air, but it must be guarded against cold, for an ordinary cold, at this stage, may quickly lead to pneumonia. A visit to the seashore, if it does not involve a long journey, and the weather is fine, is an excellent means of hastening convalescence.

In the absence of a definite cure for the disease, the treatment of whooping cough is a battle with symptoms and complications, and these are so numerous and so various in their manifestations that it is impossible to give general advice. A severe case taxes the ingenuity and experience of a specialist, and so it is apparent that the home treatment, so often depended upon, is highly dangerous. As soon as your child develops a bad cough, send for a physician; and do not grow impatient if he fails to make an immediate diagnosis and give the patient instant relief. As I have said, it is often difficult to detect whooping cough during the first week. It is possible, indeed, for a child to have the disease and yet never whoop, and it is possible, again, for a child to whoop, and yet not have a whooping cough. A child who has once had the malady is very apt to whoop for years afterward, whenever it takes cold.

Cleanliness and fresh air are just as important in the treatment of whooping cough as they are in measles or pneumonia. Let the room in which the patient is confined be cheerful and sunny, and whenever possible give it two rooms, so that one may be cleaned and disinfected while the other is in use. If the weather is fine and it is strong enough, it should be taken out for an airing every day. But if the air is damp, or there is a wind, it would best be kept indoors.

The complication most to be feared, during the winter months, is pneumonia. During the summer, particularly if the patient is very young, there is almost equal danger for diarrhea. In order to ward off the latter it is necessary to exercise great care in the diet. The patient's meals should have diluted milk and egg-albumen for their mainstays, and there should be no feeding of raw fruits or red meats, save with the consent of the physician. Among infants convulsions are not infrequent, and often they cause death. Despite the appalling fight for breath during the paroxysms of coughing, it is seldom that a patient dies by actual suffocation.

Whooping cough is such a contagious malady, and runs such a long course that it is never safe to keep other children under the same roof with a patient. As soon as the disease is detected, let the other children be sent away at once to some house in which they will be the only youngsters, and keep them away from school for sixteen days. If, at the end of that time, they appear to be in good health, they may be sent back to school.

All of these precautions are necessary because there is good reason to believe that whooping cough is contagious, not only during the whooping stage, but also in the very earliest stage. Thus a child who seems at the moment to have nothing worse than a mild cold may yet spread whooping cough from end to end of a large school. Where a hundred children are exposed to the infection, it is not uncommon for 90 to develop the disease. It is, indeed, one of the most virulent of childhood's plagues, and as I have shown, one of the most dangerous. In the United States today, it kills more children each year than scarlet fever.

The room in which a patient sleeps should be disinfected every ten days. In order that this may be done, of course, the patient must be moved to another room. As soon as all is in readiness swab the furniture with a weak solution of bichloride of mercury or carbolic acid. Then close the room tightly and burn a formaldehyde candle. After an hour or so, throw open the windows, and let the fumes of the formaldehyde escape. If this is done early in the morning, it is usually possible for a child to sleep in the room that night.

The virtue of this disinfection lies in the fact that a child recovering from whooping cough sometimes seems to become reinfected, probably from the bed-clothes or other furnishings. In other words, the patient apparently acquires the disease all over again, when on the road to recovery. Disinfection minimizes this danger, and in addition it disposes of all the stray germs that may have wandered in and so reduces the danger of pneumonia and other complications.

It is not wise to let the patient come into contact with other children until at least a month after the whooping has ceased. Even then, it is best that it sleep alone for another month. Before the rooms in which it has been housed while ill are used by other children they must be disinfected in a thorough manner. This may be done with the antiseptic solutions and the formaldehyde, using both more freely than in the periodic disinfections, but it is advisable, whenever possible, to have the work done by experts. In all large cities the health department will send men to do it, sometimes for a small fee and sometimes without charge.

There are dozens of patented remedies for whooping cough and all of them now bear the misleading notice "Guaranteed under the Pure Food and Drug Act." The layman fancies that this notice signifies, in some mysterious manner, that the national government endorses the extravagant claims of the makers. As a matter of fact, it does nothing of the sort. All it proves is that the nostrum contains no more of certain specified poisons than is indicated on the label. Innumerable drugs which, under the law, need not be specified on the label, are extremely dangerous.

It may be stated with all due fairness to the patent medicine men, that not one of their cough syrups and elixirs is of value in whooping cough. True enough, some of them may contain drugs which, in the hands of a competent physician, may be of appreciable service, but all of these do far more harm than good if the dosage is not adapted to the peculiar needs of the individual patient, and all of them are very apt to upset the stomach. Vomiting and diarrhea are common enough in whooping cough as it is. Drugs in the stomach are always foes of an uneventful recovery, and the physician, when he gives them at all, does so with great care and great reluctance.

The common home remedies are even worse than the drug-store messes. Those ghastly infusions of camomile and other herbs, so often prescribed by wise old grandmothers to provoke perspiration, and so "sweat out the fever," are the advance agents of pneumonia. So are all the ancient plasters and poultices of the family medicine chest. Let them be anathema!

I sometimes think, indeed, that the degree of civilization of a community may be judged by the contents of its average family medicine chest. In the old days this chest bulged with herbs, barks, roots, soothing syrups, headache powders, lint, salves and ointments. Paregoric was in the place of honor, and behind it stood carboys of arnica and sweet spirits of nitre.

In the future, I fancy, the medicine chest will be smaller and less horrifying. It will contain a box of aseptic cotton, a bottle of carbolic Vaseline, a bottle of castor oil, a hot water bag and very little else.

Commentary

Chapter 13: Whooping Cough: It Kills More Children than Scarlet Fever and Diphtheria Together

This chapter presents as good a description of the onset and course of whooping cough as can be found in either the popular or medical literature of the time. Whooping cough, or pertussis, is transmitted by respiratory droplets expelled into the air, usually by a cough, not unlike tuberculosis. Although pertussis is distressing and exhausting to the patient as well as his parents, it was the risk of secondary infections that made it one of the leading causes of infant mortality in 1910. Before the advent of petussis vaccine, 1 out of 4 infants under the age of 1 year who contracted whooping cough died. Pneumonia led the list of fatal complications. Treatment of pneumonia was largely supportive and it was a major cause of death in the very young, the elderly, and those too debilitated to fight it off without the aid of antibiotics.

In 1900 two French researchers at the Pasteur Institute, Jules Bordet and Octave Gengou, discovered the organism that caused whooping cough, now called *Bordetella pertussis* (after Bordet). It was not until 1906 that the Frenchmen published their results; it took them six arduous years to devise a method of growing the organism on artificial media and to fulfill all of Robert Koch's strict postulates of the germ theory.[1] One of the few inaccuracies in *What You Ought to Know About Your Baby,* in the context of the times, lies in the statement "We are yet somewhat in the dark as to the cause of whooping cough"—the pertussis organism was identified four years before the book's publication.

Once Bordet and Gengou described *Bordetella pertussis* (then referred to as *Hemophilus pertussis*), the search for a whooping cough vaccine began. By 1938, this objective was achieved. Today, the pertussis vaccine is combined with the diphtheria and tetanus toxoid vaccines and is administered to infants (infants are most susceptible to the serious complications of whooping cough) at ages 2, 4, and 6 months, with "booster" immunizations given at age 18 months and 5 years. A great deal of controversy surrounds the pertussis vaccine because the type used in most countries today, including the United States, is a "whole cell" preparation of *Bordetella pertussis*. This means that a great many elements, other than those that induce specific immunity to the microbe, appear in the vaccine. These unneeded but difficult-to-separate-out elements are also responsible for the vaccine's numerous side effects. Most of the adverse reactions to the pertussis vaccine are minor; they include local swelling, redness, and tenderness at the site of the injection, low-grade fever, and "fussiness." The majority of these minor reactions can be avoided by giving the infant a dose of acetaminophen (Tylenol) just before administering the immunization.[2]

Severe adverse effects to the pertussis vaccine are extremely rare (1/100,000), and, although they do not warrant the risk of leaving the child unimmunized, they should be mentioned: focal neurologic signs such as seizures occurring within 7 days of immunization, a shock-like state, severe allergic reactions with difficulty breathing, fevers as high as 105°F (40.5°C) within 24 hours after immunization unexplained by another cause, and brain damage. Any such adverse reactions contraindicate further use of the vaccine in that particular child. Although this list of horrors is enough to keep a mother from bringing her child to see the pediatrician, the risk of contracting whooping cough without the vaccine is 1 in 3000; the risk of permanent neurological disease from the vaccine is 1 in 300,000. Whooping cough is still a serious infection, especially for infants, with a death rate of 1% and a brain damage rate of 0.5%: that is, 1 in 100 infants with whooping cough die; 1 in 200 infants with the disease develop some form of brain damage or neurological impairment.[3-5]

It is precisely because of these complications that many public health experts and the American Academy of Pediatrics have concluded that "the risk of suffering and death caused by whooping cough is far greater than the possible side effects of the vaccine."[6] The only children who should not receive the pertussis vaccine are those who have experienced a serious adverse reaction from the vaccine, or who have epilepsy or evolving neurologic disease.

Currently, physicians, immunologists, and epidemiologists are at work evaluating an "acellular" pertussis vaccine, similar to one presently used in Japan. Acellular vaccine consists primarily of elements called hemagglutinins, which provide long-term immunity to whooping cough, but contains none of the elements that cause the potential side effects of the whole-cell pertussis vaccine.[7,8] Although it has been used with great success in children in Japan and Sweden, acellular pertussis vaccine is currently undergoing the extensive testing and field trials required by the U.S. Food and Drug Administration (F.D.A.) before it is approved for use in American infants and children. This process is an extremely slow and arduous one and requires repetition of many of the Japanese trials as well as some new ones, but it ensures that once the acellular pertussis vaccine is approved by the F.D.A. it is deemed safe as well as effective.

The chapter concludes with a reiteration of the importance of the quarantine, advice on nursing the child stricken with whooping cough, and a recurring theme in the book—the avoidance of patent medicines and folk remedies. The warning about patent medicines was repeated for good reason. For example, in 1910, the cough syrups a mother might use for her child with whooping cough contained an alarmingly large amount of opium and alcohol and had a far greater potential for harm than good. And while one of the reasons H.L. Mencken's writing is so much fun to read is the accuracy with which he predicts what the species "Boobus americanus" will do in the future, he fails dismally in predicting that the medicine chest of the future will become "smaller and less horrifying." Americans continue to rely on the modern-day equivalents of patent medicines—remedies whose efficacy has not been proved. As medicine has advanced, so has the public's demand for cures for its ailments, and the average medicine chest has increased in size over the years to accommodate them. A quick survey of the medicine chest of the first author of *The H.L. Mencken Baby Book,* he is ashamed to admit, confirms such a statement; it contains seven expired prescription medications, six different pain relievers, five cold remedies, four brands of antacids, three types of laxatives, a box of cotton swabs, a jar of Vaseline, and an old toothbrush! Mr. Mencken might complain that the preceding litany sounds like a Christmas carol for the hypochondriac.

QUESTIONS FOR THE MOTHER ABOUT CHAPTER 13

1. Why should whooping cough be especially avoided?

1910 Because the mortality is very high, especially among very young children. Babies who have whooping cough are more likely to develop pneumonia in the winter time and diarrhea in the summer time. Tuberculosis often results from the physical debility caused by whooping cough.

2. Should a child with whooping cough be isolated?

1910 Yes. Whooping cough is so exceedingly contagious that it is not safe to have other children in the same house with a whooping cough patient.

3. Should a child with whooping cough be allowed to go to school?

1910 No. One case of whooping cough can infect a school from end to end. Though children with whooping cough are able to run about, they should be kept away from all other children.

4. What is the best way to get rid of whooping cough?

1910 The room in which the child sleeps should be disinfected every ten days. Whooping cough is so exceedingly infectious that the child can reinfect itself, thus prolonging the disease. Sheets, bedding and clothes should be soaked in carbolic acid solution; woodwork and floors and walls should be washed down with this solution, and a formaldehyde candle burned every ten days.

5. Is it necessary to have a doctor for whooping cough?

1910 By all means. It is not safe to use any home remedies or patent medicines. Let the doctor watch the little patient very closely. A child with whooping cough should be warmly clothed, but should have plenty of fresh air.

REFERENCES

1. Rosen G. Acute communicable diseases. *In* Bett WR. *The History and Conquest of Common Diseases*. Norman, Oklahoma: University of Oklahoma Press, 1954, pp. 61–63. The original article by Bordet and Gengou appeared in *Annales de l'Institute Pasteur* 20:731–741, 1906.
2. Lewis K, Cherry JD, et al. The effect of prophylactic acetaminophen administration on reactions to DTP vaccination. *American Journal of Diseases of Children* 142:62–65, 1988.
3. Schmitt B. *Your Child's Health*. New York: Bantam Books, 1987, pp. 177–178.
4. Hinman AR, Koplan JP. Pertussis and pertussis vaccine: reanalysis of benefits, risks, and costs. *Journal of the American Medical Association* 251:3109–3113, 1984.
5. Cody CL, Baraff LJ, Cherry JD, *et al*. Nature and rates of adverse reactions associated with the DTP and DT immunizations in infants and children. *Pediatrics* 68:650–660, 1981.
6. Report of the Committee on Infectious Diseases: The 1986 Red Book (20th ed.). Evanston, IL: American Academy of Pediatrics, 1986, pp. 269–275.
7. Sato Y, Kimura M, Fukumi H. Development of a pertussis component vaccine in Japan. *Lancet* 1:122–126, 1984.
8. Blennow M, Granstrom M, Jaatmaa E, Olin P. Primary immunization of infants with an acellular pertussis vaccine in a double-blind randomized clinical trial. *Pediatrics* 82:293–299, 1988.

14
If Your Baby Had Pneumonia

The sinister distinction of holding first place upon the American table of mortality belongs to pneumonia, a disease of the lungs. It causes more than one-tenth of all the deaths that occur in the United States each year. It slays the babe of a few months and the grandfather of fourscore years. It lays low the rich and the poor, the sturdy and the weak, the overfed and the starving. And it is one of the few diseases that the modern physician can do little to combat. When the patient gets well, it is nearly always nature that works the cure—nature and, be it added, good nursing.

In view of this fact it is plain that every American mother should endeavor to learn something about the malady, for it is upon her, when the patient is a child, that the burden of nursing commonly falls.

Reduced to its elementals, pneumonia is nothing more than a clogging up of the lungs, due to the presence and activity of countless hordes of some breed or other of virulent germ.

As every one knows, oxygen enters the body through the nostrils and the windpipe, as a result of the act of breathing. At its lower end the windpipe divides into two branches—the bronchial tubes—one of which makes off to the right and the other to the left. At the end of each bronchial tube there is a further division, and at the end of each division another one, and so on. The incoming oxygen, proceeding down these constantly dividing passages, comes at last to the ultimate lung-cells.

Now, when virulent germs invade the lungs, the blood and tissues make an effort to paralyze and kill them, and the result of the battle is a mass of débris—dead germs, broken-off lung cells, mucous, dead blood-cells and other things. This débris fills many of the lung-cells and puts thousands of them out of commission. In consequence the blood gets less oxygen than it should get, and the heart tries to make up for the deficiency by pumping blood into the remaining clear cells a good deal faster than usual, and by making the lungs breathe faster. This plan works very well for a while, and if the blood makes good progress in killing the invading germs and the débris is quickly absorbed or coughed up, the difficulty will be tided over and the lungs will soon be working normally again. But sometimes so many cells are clogged up that the blood can not get enough oxygen, no matter how hard the heart works, and then there is great danger of collapse and death. Again, the germs may send out poisons which paralyze the heart, and then there is great danger, too. All this proves, you will observe, that pneumonia, though a lung disease, makes its final onslaught upon the heart.

The foremost pathologists in the world have been trying for many years to discover some germs specific for pneumonia, but so far their efforts have been in vain. That is to say, there is nothing under the sun that will directly kill the germs or directly aid the blood in its war upon them. It is possible, of course, to assist nature by combating the fever which appears with the disease. What the patient most needs is a clean bed and plenty of air. Given these things and a good constitution, the blood will fight the germs, rout them, kill them and get rid of them. The chances are always in favor of recovery.

An attack of pneumonia begins in a manner which suggests a very bad cold. The patient has a chill and a fever and suffers from pains in the side. A cough soon appears and the breath becomes short and quick. The valiant battle of the overworked heart is indicated by a quick pulse and flushed cheeks. Soon there are signs of great exhaustion, with headache, sleeplessness and (sometimes) delirium.

During all of this period the blood is waging a tremendous war upon the invading germs. If it is destined to lose, the exhaustion will grow more and more marked and the patient will die. But if it is destined to win there will come a time—it will be between the fifth and the tenth day—when the patient will suddenly seem brighter. The temperature will fall, the breathing will be more regular, and the violent jumping of the pulse will cease. When this happens it is a sign that the battle is won.

But though the germs have been conquered, it is just at this stage that careful nursing is most needed. The lungs are full of purulent wreckage, and the business of getting rid of this is difficult. The attack itself has greatly exhausted the patient, and his strength is next to nothing. Good nursing must recruit it for him—nursing which takes the form of plenty of fresh air and a supply of easily assimilated food.

The fact that pneumonia might be called simply a shutting-off of oxygen shows how important it is to give the patient plenty of air. In several large New York hospitals, indeed, sufferers from the disease are carried to the roof, and kept there day and night. When your child grows ill, move it to the largest and sunniest room in the house, and open the windows. If it is too cold for that, have another room near by, into which the patient may be moved at least three times a day, to permit a thorough ventilation of the sick-room. All unnecessary furniture and all pictures, hangings and other impediments should be taken out of both rooms.

It is dangerous to permit pneumonia patients to remain too long in one position. They should be moved about often, and should be frequently propped up with pillows. The notion that the child must be buried in blankets to protect it from "catching cold" is little more than a mere superstition. The child already has the worst of all conceivable colds, and what it needs, beyond everything else, is air and freedom of movement.

When the little patient's temperature ranges alarmingly high, some means should be employed to bring this temperature down, but this means should never take the form of drugs. The use of such things as phenacetine, antipyrin, acetanilid and their combinations is exceedingly hazardous, on account of their interference with the proper working of the heart. Quinine is almost as bad. The best thing to do is to sponge the baby with alcohol or cold water. Next after that comes the use of icebags and compresses.

During the bath it is a good plan to rub the child's skin all over—of course, very gently. This has a good effect upon the circulation, and tends to prevent delirium and restlessness. In addition, there is probably some more subtle psychic effect. Every one knows how pleasant it is to be gently massaged—how it drives away pain, calms the nerves and produces a feeling of healthfulness and well-being. Sleep and comparative comfort usually follow the bath and rubbing down. Upon the reappearance of any nervous symptoms, repeat the bath.

As I have said, it is impossible to aid the body directly in its struggle with the pneumonia organisms, but there are countless ways of giving it indirect assistance. When a cough is severe, for example, a good effect is often produced by the inhalation of the vapors of creosote, carbolic acid or menthol. Again, alcohol and other stimulants are often capable of lending the heart a hand at a critical moment. But it is not well for the mother to employ such things on her own responsibility. Have the doctor give you full instructions, and then carry them out faithfully.

There are so many varieties of pneumonia that it would be impossible to specify all of them. What is known as broncho-pneumonia is the most common form among small children. Six times out of ten it appears as a sequel to whooping cough or some other infantile ailment, and is then usually traceable to faulty nursing. It represents, indeed, nothing more than a transfer of the germ of some disease to the lungs.

True lobar pneumonia usually comes on suddenly, like a bolt from the blue, and not as a sequel of some other malady. It is most common between the ages of three and eight and usually attacks children who have seemed to be perfectly healthy. It always follows the course I have described, whereas bronchial pneumonia may drag on for weeks, and in some cases may become genuinely chronic. The immediate death-rate in lobar pneumonia is higher than in the bronchial variety, but, in the long run, it is less to be dreaded, for it is seldom marked by relapses, and recovery, when it occurs, is always complete.

After a child has had pneumonia, no matter what form of the malady, and convalescence has begun, it is best to take it to the country. The disease leaves the body enormously thirsty for fresh air; and fresh air, in a large city, is almost a curiosity. Besides that, a change of scene is always of great benefit during recovery. Unluckily, pneumonia confers no durable immunity. As a matter of fact, the recovered patient is more liable to the disease than it was before the attack. In addition, its weakened lungs afford unusually good soil for the germs of other maladies, too, and one of these is tuberculosis. Fresh air is the only thing that can reduce this liability.

At times, pneumonia sweeps through an entire household, and in all cases it is well to isolate the patient, particularly when there are other children in the house. Your own child may be protected against pneumonia by very simple precautions. See that it gets wholesome, easily digested food and that it has plenty of air, day and night. Too much coddling is the principal cause of childish ailments.

You may think that fresh air causes colds, but as a matter of fact the very reverse is true. The child that is always taking cold is the child who has been coddled and whose mode of life ill adapts it to meeting the vicissitudes of existence here on earth. It is part of life for all of us, now and then, to stand in drafts and to get our feet wet. No matter how much we try to avoid it, we must do so at frequent intervals. Therefore, the thing to do with a child is, not to make a vain attempt to protect it against accidental and inevitable exposure, but so to rear it that it will be able to face such exposure without damage. A cold is always a sign of a low power of resistance. The entirely healthy human being never takes cold.

Therefore, when your baby begins to cough and snuffle, send for your doctor and have him examine it. The very fact that it is coughing is proof that it needs attention. The doctor's visit, if it is made in time, may head off an attack of pneumonia. Most mothers regard a cold as a trivial and harmless thing, but, as I have shown, it is not. The difference between a cold and pneumonia is one of degree only, and not one of kind. Both are definite infections, and both prove, with equal force, that the little patient is not as well fitted as he should be to survive in the struggle for existence.

In conclusion, let me warn all mothers who read this chapter to remember that there is no reason for flying into a panic when the doctor's verdict is "pneumonia." Given good and faithful nursing and obedience to the doctor's orders, there is no reason why your child should not get well. In all cases, no matter how serious, the chances are in favor of recovery.

Commentary

Chapter 14: If Your Baby Had Pneumonia

Mencken and Hirshberg's essay on pneumonia is a superb and articulate description of an extremely deadly illness that was responsible for more than 10% of all deaths in the United States in 1910 alone. Pneumonia was deemed by pediatricians as "the most important factor in the mortality of infancy and childhood."[1] Internists also had a great deal of respect for the consequences of pneumonia. Sir William Osler, for example, referred to the disease as "the present captain of the men of death."[2] It was for this reason that many a physician and nurse referred to pneumonia as "the old man's friend"; elderly, debilitated patients would frequently develop pneumonia and die from the infection in a rather peaceful manner. Mencken, too, graphically describes pneumonia as a widespread and indiscriminate killer of those of all ages and all stations of life: "It slays the babe of a few months and the grandfather of fourscore years. It lays low the rich and the poor, the sturdy and the weak, the overfed and the starving." Further, pneumonia was a feared complication of other diseases, such as measles, whooping cough, and scarlet fever, and it could easily bring about a rapid death once it appeared.

Although this essay presents an accurate description of the pathology of pneumonia, these concepts took physicians from Hippocrates (460–370 B.C.) to R.T.H. Laennec (1781–1826) and Carl von Rokitansky (1804–1878) over 2000 years to sort out.[3] Our understanding of pneumonia evolved in concert with the underlying medical concepts of each era. Hippocrates, the Father of Medicine, explained pneumonia as an imbalance of the humors and treated the condition empirically by bleeding the patient. As theories of solidism began to develop in the early 18th century, physicians tried to correlate specific diseases with specific locations or "seats" in the organs. Observant physicians who performed their own autopsies, such as the Dutch clinician Hermann Boerhaave in 1709, noted the gross lung changes of pneumonia described in this chapter. Clinicians of the French school, specifically René Théophile Hyacinthe Laennec, used this information to develop reliable means of clinical observation and diagnosis for conditions such as pneumonia, pulmonary tuberculosis, and other lung diseases. Laennec's technique of tapping on a patient's chest, or percussion, to distinguish normal, air-filled lungs from dull-sounding, fluid-filled lungs, and his invention of the stethoscope in 1819 for the study of a patient's breath sounds greatly advanced our ability to diagnose pneumonia. The study of pneumonia was particularly advanced by Carl von Rokitansky who, in 1849, distinguished the specific types of pneumonia using a microscope. The advent of x-rays in 1895 allowed physicians to noninvasively visualize a patient's lungs infected with pneumonia. It was finally the bacteriologists, proponents of the germ theory, who discovered bacterial causes of the various types of pneumonia seen by clinicians, setting the stage for the antibiotic revolution of the mid-20th century.

Despite the marked improvement in the understanding of the pathophysiology of pneumonia and its diagnosis, treatment of the illness well into the 1920s seems shocking and barbaric by today's standards. Profuse bleeding of the patient was a standard method of treating pneumonia during the 1920s. George Orwell, the British author and essayist, recalled being treated for pneumonia in 1929 with wet-cupping, a means of withdrawing blood from an incision, in a Paris hospital. Other treatment modalities included the administration of copious amounts of fluids (probably the best form of treatment available), expectorants that induced salivation, injections of stimulants such as digitalis and strychnine, strong purgatives that emptied the bowels, brandy, oxygen, hypnotics, and sedatives.[4] The treatment of choice, however, as detailed by Mencken and Hirshberg, and testified to in scores of medical reports, was good nursing care, close observation, making the patient as comfortable as possible, and a tincture of time.

The authors also describe a phenomenon of pneumonia that is rarely seen today: the crisis. Without antibiotic treatment, pneumonia rapidly progresses and the patient becomes weaker and more debilitated, often exhausted by the high fevers and labored breathing that are hallmarks of untreated pneumonia. The crisis of pneumonia refers to whether or not the patient would win the "tremendous war" his immune system waged "upon the invading germs." The very young, the old and extremely ill, and malnourished alcoholics, among others, frequently lost this battle. The remainder of patients with pneumonia, seemingly at death's door, would miraculously become better 10 to 14 days after the onset of symptoms, much to the surprise and joy of their physicians. Dr. Lewis Thomas, in his memoirs of internship and residency at the Boston City Hospital, referred to his patients' victories over the crisis of pneumonia as one of the most gratifying events he ever witnessed.[5]

In 1884, the German bacteriologist Albert Frankel discovered that the bacterial organism *Streptococcus pneumoniae* was the leading cause of community-acquired pneumonia, although any number of bacterial and viral agents can cause a similar infection in the lungs. Other important factors that can make a person more susceptible to a particular type of pneumonia include whether or not the patient had a preexisting infection such as measles, whooping cough, or a severe illness; the age and general health of the patient; and whether the pneumonia was acquired in a hospital or in the community. The latter factor is important because hospitals are frequently colonized with hearty, highly resistant organisms that rarely cause disease in healthy individuals but are a real threat to those who are significantly ill. Fortunately, cupping devices, cauteries, and the cathartics formerly used to treat pneumonia have been relegated to medical museums; the development and refinement of antibiotics have made the management of pneumonia relatively routine.

QUESTIONS FOR THE MOTHER ABOUT CHAPTER 14

1. What is the one preventive as well as cure for pneumonia?
1910   Fresh air.

2. How will fresh air cure pneumonia?

1910 Pneumonia is a disease that shuts off oxygen from the lungs. Therefore the patient needs to get as much fresh air as possible. Its bed should be put on the piazza or roof or under a large window.

3. How will fresh air prevent pneumonia?

1910 It builds up the body, makes a child hardy, and its blood able to resist cold and pneumonia germs. Keep the children out of doors all day. Let them sleep in the open air at night and do not worry about pneumonia.

4. Why should a cold be treated as if it were the most serious of diseases?

1910 Because it is a sign that the child is run down; that its body is in a condition to be attacked by other germs. Because a cold neglected may lead to pneumonia or even tuberculosis. Because a cold is often a symptom of a contagious disease. If the child is not isolated, the family or school may be exposed to contagion.

5. Why should a child with a cold have a thorough physical examination by a doctor?

1910 Not only that he may prevent the cold from developing into something more serious, but because it is a sign that the child needs a change of air, of food or habits. It is often a sign that the child has adenoids, and adenoids may open the way for pneumonia or tuberculosis.

6. Why should a pneumonia patient have the constant care of a physician and a graduate nurse?

1910 Because the death rate from pneumonia is very great and is constantly increasing; because the disease is so severe and short. Three, two or even one day may decide whether an attack of pneumonia means life or death.

7. What care should a convalescent have?

1910 He should have his lungs thoroughly examined, have a "culture" taken to be sure he has not tuberculosis. He should take pains to avoid fatigue, over-heated rooms; should make a point of eating plenty of nourishing food, and of keeping out in the fresh air.

REFERENCES

1. Holt LE. *Diseases of Childhood and Infancy* (3rd ed.). New York: D. Appleton and Co., 1907, p. 525.
2. Cushing H. *The Life of Osler,* Vol 1. Oxford: Oxford University Press, 1977, p. 553. Actually Osler borrowed the phrase from the British writer and preacher John Bunyan who, in 1680, called tuberculosis "the captain of these men of death."
3. Brockbank EM, Brockbank W. Pneumonia. *In* Bett WR (ed.). *The History and Conquest of Common Diseases.* Norman, Oklahoma: University of Oklahoma Press, 1954, pp.84–98.
4. Ibid, pp. 94–95.
5. Thomas L. *The Youngest Science.* New York: The Viking Press. 1983, pp. 41–44.

15
Need Every Child Have Measles?

Next to the common cold, measles is probably the most wide-spread of all infectious diseases, at least in civilized countries. Almost everyone gets over it, many do not. This has led to the popular idea that measles is something to be regarded lightly, and that it is best, all things considered, for a child to take it and have it over. Nothing could be further from the truth. In itself, perhaps measles is seldom a direct cause of death, but too often it leaves the body in a very debilitated state, and other, and worse, maladies come in its train. Thus, like influenza, it is chiefly to be feared, not on its own account, but on account of the things that follow it.

No one has yet succeeded in tracking down, with certainty, the germ that causes measles. We know that the cause is a germ, because its effects and mode of multiplication are exactly those of other germs, but beside the fact that it is an animal parasite we know very little else about it. Until we learn more, it will be impossible to make a direct war upon it. Even now, of course, we can take measures to prevent its spread from one person to another, and after it has begun its work we can deal with symptoms and complications it produces, but we know of no way to kill it, once it has invaded the body, and we know of no way to limit or modify its activity there.

Fortunately for us, nature knows more than we do. As soon as the measles germ enters the body, nature begins to battle with it, and in the vast majority of cases she succeeds in stamping it out. This battle is begun automatically, and—unless death intervenes—it always proceeds in a more or less regular manner. In consequence we say that measles is a self-limiting disease, which means that it runs a clearly-marked course, beginning with the first appearance of the germs in the body and ending with their complete destruction and expulsion.

The more obvious signs of measles—the fever, the lassitude, the sore eyes, running nose, and sore throat, and beyond all, the red rash—are familiar to every one. There are, in addition, several signs which give earlier warning, but which are seldom perceptible, save to the physician. One of them is Koplik's sign, so called after the New York pathologist who first noticed it. It consists in the appearance of small blue-white specks on the mucous membrane lining the inside of the cheeks. These specks usually appear two or three days before the rash and so they give the physician a chance to be forewarned and forearmed. They explain why it is that when a child complains of feeling ill and shows a rising fever, the doctor usually makes a thorough examination of its mouth.

After a child has been exposed to measles, it takes from eleven to fourteen days for the disease to develop. The first symptom is a general feeling of illness and uneasiness, with the signs, perhaps, of a bad cold in the head. Then the eyes begin to water, the temperature rises, the throat becomes sore, there is a cough, and on the third or fourth day the characteristic eruption appears. As a rule, it is first seen along the edge of the hair—on the forehead or neck, or behind the ears. It is made up of small, dark-red spots, often some distance apart and flat with the skin. These spots soon begin to swell and multiply, and in a short while the whole face is covered with them and they begin to appear on the neck and chest, and so on down to the feet. By the time they reach the feet, they are commonly beginning to dry up upon the face. Usually they are in groups, with areas of clear skin between, but sometimes they cover the face so thickly that scarcely a speck of clear skin is to be seen. At such times, the whole face is swelled and the eyes are almost closed.

There are three or four days of this, and then the little pustules begin to grow pale and dry. This is the period of desquamation, or shedding. The dead skin breaks off into small scales, much resembling bran, and the new skin begins to appear underneath. In scarlet fever the skin comes off in large patches, but in measles the scales are small. Often, indeed, they are so small that they are scarcely noticed.

This shedding continues, as a rule, from five to ten days, though occasionally it may be prolonged to two weeks. It is accompanied by annoying itching, and there is commonly some cough too, and a lingering weakness in the eyes, but otherwise the patient begins to feel perfectly well again. The appetite returns, the fever has abated, and, if all has gone well, there is nothing amiss in throat or lungs.

Sometimes the rash in measles is so severe that the small blood vessels in the skin are broken down, and the blood in them comes out. The blood collects under the surface of the skin in small dark patches, much as in a bruise or black eye. This condition was described by the older doctors as "black measles," and it was believed that death almost invariably followed. But, as a matter of fact, the appearance of these dark spots need not cause a panic. As a rule, true enough, they indicate a case worse than the average, but they have been noted, also, in comparatively mild cases, and in themselves they do no harm. It often happens that a few such hemorrhagic eruptions appear in the course of an ordinary case.

As I have said, nothing can be done to *cure measles,* as we can cure malaria, diphtheria or a broken arm. The disease must run its course, and we can never even tell how long that course is going to be, save very roughly. But it is perfectly possible to guard the little patient against the disastrous complications which lurk along the trail of the measles germ, and it is possible, too, to relieve much of the patient's suffering. In accomplishing this, the nurse plays a part more important perhaps than that of the doctor.

As soon as a child grows ill and feverish, and begins to complain of discomfort in the eyes and nasal passages, it should be put to bed in a well-ventilated, darkened room, and the physician should be summoned. So many infantile maladies begin in the same way that it is often impossible, at this stage, to say whether the little patient is developing measles, scarlet fever, influenza, or merely a cold, but it is always best, whenever it shows a fever, however slight, to put it to bed. In a day or two, more certain diagnosis will follow the first doubt.

Let me say here with all possible emphasis, that putting a child to bed does not mean burying it beneath a matterhorn of woolen blankets. There is a popular notion, that, in all maladies accompanied by fever, a vigorous and constant perspiration is beneficial and necessary, but this is scarcely true. Sweating will not modify the course of measles, and neither will bad air, except in an unfavorable way. See that the patient is well protected from all draughts, but let the blankets be light enough for comfort, and make sure that there is constant ingress of fresh air into the room.

As a help toward that sweating which woolen blankets, however thick, only partly achieve, it is customary, among amateur nurses, to employ vast doses of various hot teas. All such disgusting messes should be thrown to the dogs. Camomile, sassafras or what-not—they do a lot of harm and no good at all. It is difficult to make the average grandmother believe that camomile is a fraud, and so, when she recommends it and you refuse to administer it, she will go away offended, but it is far better to offend her than to injure your child. All the little patient needs, in the way of drink, is plenty of cooled water—not ice water, but water of the ordinary hydrant temperature. Do not keep a pitcher full in the sick-room, but draw a fresh glass of a pure or boiled water that has been cooled whenever it is wanted. Day or night, never deny the child a drink.

Regarding the food to be given to the patient, it is best to consult the attending physician in the particular instance. In an ordinary case of measles, the child will be satisfied with milk, soft-boiled eggs and meat broths during its few days of severe illness, and may approach its usual diet soon thereafter, but in case there are complications, particularly in the digestive tract, great care in feeding must be exercised. Have the doctor draw up a bill of fare and fix the meal times, and then stick to the schedule religiously. A feverish child requires very little food and it is best never to try to force it to eat.

The patient's eyes will probably be inflamed and painful. Keep them clean by swabbing them every few hours with a little mop of sterilized cotton that has been dipped into a solution of boracic acid. The cotton comes in boxes to be had for ten cents or a quarter at any drug store. Never use ordinary raw cotton, for no matter how clean it may seem, it is always full of irritating particles and the germs of various diseases. The boracic acid is a near relative to borax and may be had at the drug store. Put a tablespoonful into a tumbler of water and use the clear solution.

If there is so much discharge from the eyes that the lids stick together, dip a piece of the sterilized cotton into Vaseline and gently smear the edges of the lids. Sometimes the eyes are so painful and so much inflamed that it is necessary to apply ice-packs to them. When this is necessary, the doctor will show you how to do it.

There is a great deal of itching in measles, particularly after the dead skin begins to shed. To relieve it, apply a thin film of Vaseline—either the plain or the carbolated. Besides reducing the itching, this will loosen the scales and so help the process of desquamation. But never rub the skin! The friction of the washrag or cotton and the clothing is all that nature needs.

During the few days of fever, of course, the child need be bathed only at the doctor's orders. As soon as the shedding begins it should have a daily warm bath. This should be given with the room warm and all the windows closed, and it should not be prolonged. Use a very soft washcloth or absorbent cotton and little, if any, soap; and after drying, anoint all those parts of the body upon which the rash has appeared with Vaseline. The physician may prescribe some other ointment, but if he does not it is best to use only Vaseline. The common drug store salves and ointments may do a great deal of harm.

The child's cough, headache, sore throat and other discomforts must be combatted, not by the nurse, but by the physician. Aside from its simple food and its plentiful supply of cooled water, it should take nothing into its stomach that has not been prescribed by its medical attendant. There are dozens of grandmothers' elixirs for the various symptoms of measles, and all of them are abominations. From boneset tea to sweet spirits of nitre they are dangerous frauds, one and all.

Measles is an exceedingly contagious disease, but its virulence, unlike that of scarlet fever, does not last very long. As soon as a case appears in a household, all of the other children should be kept from school, but it is unnecessary to send them out of the house. The room in which the patient is being nursed should be isolated from the rest of the house, with as rigid a quarantine as if the contagion was always fatal. If the mother is the nurse, she should keep away from the other children until at least two weeks after the patient has recovered. It is possible for a child to take measles by merely passing the open door of a room in which a patient is confined.

If, as often happens, there are two patients at the same time, it is best, whenever possible, to put them into separate rooms. This is because the more dangerous maladies which sometimes follow or complicate measles, such as pneumonia, are apt to be communicated from one patient to another. Herein, no doubt, we find an explanation of the fact that epidemics of measles are always more severe in boarding-schools and orphan-asylums than among children at home. One patient developing pneumonia or diphtheria communicates it to many others.

Inasmuch as measles is already contagious before its outward signs appear—that is, during the period of incubation, or breeding—it is exceedingly difficult to protect a child against it, particularly if the child goes to school or to Sunday School, or otherwise associates with its fellows. But in the case of weakly children, it is well to make extraordinary efforts to secure this protection, for measles, in such children, very frequently leads to pneumonia, chronic bronchitis, and even tuberculosis. If, after an attack, the patient continues to cough and to remain weak, it should be sent into the country; preferably, to the mountains. The seeds of life-long illness and early death are sowed by apparently mild attacks of measles.

A week after the last signs of shedding have disappeared it is safe to permit the patient to mingle again with other children. But before the room in which it has been confined is used as a sleeping apartment, it should be thoroughly disinfected. The measles germs do not cling to life very vigorously, and outside of the human body they soon die, but it is well to take no chances.

Commentary

Chapter 15: Need Every Child Have Measles?

When *What You Ought to Know About Your Baby* first appeared in print, measles was the most commonly diagnosed of the childhood diseases that produce an eruptive rash (e.g., measles, German measles, chickenpox, small pox, and erythema infectiosum). The danger of the disease was not so much the rash, or the profusely watery eyes and nose, or the fever and malaise that accompanied a measles infection, but rather the potential complications that came "in its train." In this discussion on the perils of contracting measles, Mencken and Hirshberg reiterate the important concept that the patient ill with an infectious disease is far more susceptible to the ravages of other contagious processes and ill health than the normal host. Complications that were particularly feared by pediatricians in 1910 included pneumonia (which when contracted subsequent to measles had a mortality rate of 70%), ear and sinus infections, and measles encephalitis, an infection and inflammation of the brain that occurs in 1 out of 1500 cases of measles. The complications explained the death rate—4 to 5% of all cases of measles.[1] Yet relatively few pediatricians in practice today have even seen a case of measles thanks to an effective vaccine.

As noted, measles was often confused with other acute infections, particularly those that yielded some type of rash. In the medieval era, for example, measles was considered to be a less life-threatening variant of the same process that caused small pox. This erroneous theory was first proposed by the eminent Persian physician Rhazes (860–932 A.D.), one of medicine's great observers of disease, and was propagated well into the 18th century. In keeping with Rhazes' theory, small pox was termed *variolae,* Latin for the shallow pits or scars left by a small pox infection, whereas measles was referred to as *morbilli,* the diminutive of the Latin *morbus,* or deadly, indicating that measles was considered a little or mild disease in comparison to its presumed relative small pox. The English term "measles" was most likely introduced by John of Gaddesden (1280–1361), who is said to be the model for Chaucer's Doctor of Physic. At that time, the word *measles,* derived from the Latin *miselli* and *misellae,* referred to the blood-blisters or sores found on a person with leprosy. By some strange line of reasoning, John of Gaddesden connected the leprous lesions to morbilli and hence its rather interesting but inaccurate name. Eventually, the word measles lost its connection to leprosy and today is associated only with the childhood disease.[2]

Measles was confused not only with small pox but also with scarlet fever, and its diagnosis was difficult. It was the great British physician Thomas Sydenham (1624–1689) who clearly diagnosed the essential clinical features of both measles and scarlet fever, relying on the two major tenets of his theory of medicine: careful observation at the bedside and a large fund of experience. A devout follower of the Hippocratic theory of humoralism, Sydenham correctly asserted that each disease had a regular course and natural history of its own. He emphasized that each disease belonged to an individual species that could be described by the observant physician in a fashion similar to the botanist's study of plant forms. By applying this reasoning to measles and scarlet fever, he described each disease's symptoms in 1675. Measles is heralded by fever, cough, a runny nose, watery eyes that are sensitive to light, and, of course, a red, confluent, non-raised rash that begins on the face and works its way down. The rash of scarlet fever, on the other hand, or scarlatina as the British and French liked to call it, is not nearly as uniform and consists of a "goose-bumpy" rash on a base of diffusely red skin. Matters become more difficult, however, when rashes do not present in a "classic" manner, and physicians, unsure of what they are describing, invent adjectives such as morbilliform or scarlatinaform, meaning "like measles" or "like scarlet fever." Sydenham, incidentally, was one of the "older doctors" Mencken refers to who incorrectly held that hemorrhagic or "black" measles was invariably followed by death.[3,4]

Another important figure in the delineation of measles was Peter Ludwig Panum (1820–1885) who, as a 26-year-old, newly graduated medical doctor, was sent by the Danish government to the remote and isolated Faroe Islands in the North Atlantic Ocean. His mission was to investigate and study an epidemic of measles there in 1846. Just as Sydenham determined the important clinical symptoms of the disease, Panum used the Faroe Islands as a living laboratory in order to delineate the epidemiologic aspects of measles. These features, as detailed in this chapter, include the incubation period of measles, the fact that all ages are susceptible to measles but one attack confers immunity, the period when measles is most contagious (during the prodromal phase, when the patient experiences cold-like symptoms, and presence of fever prior to development of the measles rash), and the then-novel concept that measles was purely a contagious disease and isolation was the most successful means of arresting an epidemic.[5]

Although it was accepted that measles was transmitted when a susceptible person comes in close physical contact with nasopharyngeal secretions of an infected person, the etiologic agent of measles, morbillivirus, was not yet known in 1910. Further, the diagnosis of measles was a difficult matter until the characteristic measles rash erupted; by this time, however, the child was contagious to others for as long as 4 days. It was for this reason that Dr. Henry Koplik's description in 1896 of the grayish-white spots that appear on the inner lining or buccal mucosa of an infected person's mouth 3 to 4 days before the appearance of the measles rash was so important to physicians.[6] Here, at last, was a reliable and specific sign (still called Koplik's spots) obtained simply by looking into a patient's mouth and recognizing the lesions that would facilitate a confident diagnosis and early quarantine.

Measles was proved to be caused by a virus in 1911 by John F. Anderson and Joseph Goldberger. This work was greatly expanded upon by Drs. Harry Plotz, John Enders, T.C. Peebles, Samuel Katz, M.J. Milanovic, and others, who from 1938 to the early 1960s developed techniques to grow measles virus in culture. These efforts made feasible the first effective measles vaccine in 1963. Today, the measles vaccine is greater than 90–98% efficacious in providing long-term immunity against the virus. It is given in concert with the mumps and rubella vaccines at the age of 15 months. This corresponds to when the infant begins to lose the immune factors it inherited passively from its mother's blood while *in utero*. The vaccine stimulates antibody formation against the virus before actual exposure to it and has been extremely successful in the United States in nearly eradicating measles. Consider these striking figures: in 1963, before the distribution of the measles vaccine, there were 4,000,000 cases of measles, 4,000 cases of measles encephalitis, and 400 recorded deaths from complications of measles in the United States.[7] In 1983, after 20 years of providing measles vaccinations, there were less than 1500 cases of measles reported in the U.S. Measles has been slowly on the rise, however, since 1985, particularly among college-aged adolescents and young adults. For example, over 6,000 cases were reported in 1986.[8] Explanations offered for this small but significant increase in the incidence of measles includes the theorized loss of immunity or a "wearing off" effect of early batches of the vaccine, nonoptimal times of administering the vaccine, and decreasing immunization levels among preschool children. Indeed, in poor urban areas only 50% of children under 2 years of age are immunized against measles. Nationally, this figure is somewhat better; the United States Immunization Survey found that 66 to 85% of the country's 2-year-olds were immunized in 1983.

Regardless of the exact cause of the recently noted failure rate of the measles vaccine, the result is a potential effect upon the delicately balanced "herd immunity" against measles. Herd immunity means that in order to have a rapid spread of an infectious agent, a high proportion of the population in question must be susceptible to it. Epidemiologists estimate that at least 85% of the population needs to be vaccinated against measles in order to benefit from herd immunity. Any time greater than 15% of members of a community are unprotected by vaccine, an epidemic or outbreak can occur if the infectious agent enters that community.

Many public health officials and experts, such as New York State Health Commissioner Dr. David Axelrod, and Dr. Donald A. Anderson, Dean of the Johns Hopkins School of Public Health and Hygiene, have advocated a second or booster dose of measles vaccine administered between the ages of 4 and 6 years. This booster shot has been shown to greatly diminish the risk of measles and its potential complications to those 3000–5000 Americans who appear to remain susceptible to measles after receiving only one dose. The cost of the additional vaccine is about $33.00 per single shot, but the subsequent cost, both physical and financial, of an epidemic would be much higher.[9,10]

Measles remains a serious source of morbidity and mortality worldwide, especially in underdeveloped countries, where approximately 2,000,000 deaths per year are attributed to the disease and its complications. Fortunately, and in spite of imperfections in the current measles vaccine program that need to be elucidated and solved, a child with measles appearing in the emergency room of any major hospital in the United States today is rarity that would arouse the most complaisant of medical students and the sleepiest of interns.

QUESTIONS FOR THE MOTHER ABOUT CHAPTER 15

1. Why should every precaution be taken to protect a child from measles?

1910 Because though it is not often fatal, it weakens the child so that it readily takes other diseases.

2. What are the first signs of measles?

1910 A cold, fever, sore throat and weariness; later a red rash and blue-white spots inside the cheeks.

3. Why should a child with measles be quarantined?

1910 Because measles is contagious and it is not fair to other children to give them a disease that may lower their vitality and pave the way for other diseases.

4. How long should a child that has been exposed to measles be kept away from other children?

1910 It takes from eleven to fourteen days for the disease to develop.

5. What precautions should be taken to prevent the spread of measles?

1910 Measles should be reported to the Board of Health; a sign MEASLES should be put on the door. No one but the nurse should be allowed to go into the child's room or to pass the door when it is open. The room should be thoroughly fumigated before it is used again.

6. What are the special precautions to prevent bad after-effects from measles?

1910 The room should be kept dark, and the child should not be allowed to read, write or sew or to use its eyes at any close-range work. Great care should be taken that the child does not catch cold. This does not mean that all the windows should be kept closed. Fresh air in a sick-room is the best preventive of colds. The lungs and throat of a child should be thoroughly examined after measles, and it should have rest, nourishing food and outdoor life until its health is thoroughly restored.

REFERENCES

1. Holt LE. *Diseases of Childhood and Infancy*. New York: D. Appleton and Co., 1907, pp. 977–992.
2. Rosen G. Acute Communicable Diseases *In* Bett WR (ed.). *The History and Conquest of Common Diseases*. Norman, Oklahoma: University of Oklahoma Press, 1954, pp. 38–45.
3. Latham RG (Editor). *The Works of Thomas Sydenham,* Vol. 2. London: Sydenham Society, 1850, pp. 250–251.
4. Garrison FH. *An Introduction to the History of Medicine* (4th ed.). Philadelphia: WB Saunders Co., 1929.
5. Panum PL. Observations made during the epidemic of measles on the Faroe Islands in the year 1846. *Medical Classics* 3:829–886, 1939.
6. Koplik H. The diagnosis of the invasion of measles from a study of the exanthema as it appears on the buccal mucous membrane. *Archives of Pediatrics* 13:918–922, 1986.

7. Editorial. Measles, a renewed challenge. *Journal of the American Medical Association* 216:1018, 1971.

8. Markowitz LE, et al. Patterns of transmission in measles outbreaks in the United States, 1985-1986. *New England Journal of Medicine* 320:75–81, 1989.

9. Altman LK. Scientists, hoping to end measles, find a surprisingly resilient foe. *New York Times* March 28, 1989. p. C3.

10. McFadden RD. Doctors asked to give 2nd measles vaccine. *New York Times* April 30, 1989, p. 44 (section 1).

Notes

Many of the essays in the book *What You Ought to Know About Your Baby* appeared first in the *Delineator* magazine. The original references are as follows:

Chapter 1: "Slaughter of the Innocents." *Delineator* (May 1909); 73:681, 713–714.

Chapter 2: "The New-born Baby." *Delineator* (October 1908): 72:592.

Chapter 3: "The Baby's First Few Months." *Delineator* (November 1908): 72:812–813.

Chapter 4: "The Nursing Baby." *Delineator* (December 1908); 72:1014–1015.

Chapter 5: "Mother and Baby." *Delineator* (January 1909); 73:106.

Chapter 6: "The Bottle Fed Baby." *Delineator* (February 1909): 73:262–264.

Chapter 7: "A Chapter on Milk." *Delineator* (March 1909): 73:438–440.

Chapter 8: "The Food for Growing Children" appeared exclusively in the 1910 book edition of What You Ought to Know About Your Baby.

Chapter 9: "What You Ought to Know About Your School" appeared under the title "The Child Ready For School." *Delineator* (October 1909):74:327.

Chapter 10: "Need Every Child Have Catching Diseases?" appeared exclusively in the 1910 book edition of *What You Ought to Know About Your Baby*.

Chapter 11: "If Your Baby Had Diphtheria." Although there exist memoranda and editorials to suggest this article was to appear in the *Delineator,* it was never published until the book *What You Ought to Know About Your Baby* appeared.

Chapter 12: "If Your Baby Had Scarlet Fever." *Delineator* (August 1908):72:258–259, 293.

Chapter 13: "Whooping Cough: It Kills More than Diphtheria and Scarlet Fever Together" appeared exclusively in the 1910 book edition of *What You Ought to Know About Your Baby*.

Chapter 14: "If Your Baby Had Pneumonia." *Delineator* (February 1908); 72:233–234.

Chapter 15: "Need Every Child Have Measles?" appeared exclusively in the 1910 book edition of *What You Ought to Know About Your Baby*.

The only other Mencken-Hirshberg collaborations were two magazine articles that preceded the appearance of *What You Ought to Know About Your Baby* and the *Delineator* articles:

1. Hirshberg LK. Popular Medical Fallacies. *The American Magazine* (formerly *Leslie's Monthly Magazine*) (October 1906) 62:655–660.

2. Hirshberg LK. Cancer, the Unconquered Plague. The *American Magazine* (formerly *Leslie's Monthly Magazine* (February 1907) 63:374–378.

Index

ABDOMEN, of newborn infant,
    appearance of, 46
    rupture of, from excessive crying,
        56, 62
Adenoids, 30–31
    definition of, 41–42
    enlargement of, 42, 43
    removal of, 43–44
AIDS, contagiousness of, 152
AIDS epidemic, similarities to
    epidemics of old, 130–131
Alcohol, during pregnancy or
    nursing, 97
    effect on breastfeeding, 91
American Academy of Pediatrics,
    address of, 52
    Committee on Drugs of, list of
        medications that affect
        breastfeeding, 80
    Committee on Nutrition of,
        current recommendations
        for feeding infants and
        toddlers, 109–110
        recommendations about cow's
        milk, 99
    position on pertussis vaccine,
        161–162
American College of Nurse-
    Midwives, 54
American Magazine, Mencken and
    Hirshberg's collaborative
    medical writing for, 11
"Anatomical idea," 127
Anderson, John F., 181
Antibiotics, in treatment of bacterial
    infections, 41
Antitoxin, diphtheria, 133–137, 141,
    142, 143

Apnea, 43
Artificial feeding of infants. *See*
    Bottlefeeding: Formulas

BABY. *See also* Infant
    bathing of, 67, 72–73
    bouncing of, 28
    coddling of, warning against,
        33, 34
    "cost" of, 37
    kissing of, warning against, 33,
        65, 68, 70–71, 139
    rocking of, 65, 68
    what you ought to know about
        your, 27–184
        origin of book, 12–18
Bacteria, in milk, 41–42, 86–87
    infectious disease and, 41–42
Bacterial infections, management
    of, 41
Baltimore, Sage of. *See* Mencken,
    Henry Louis
Baltimore Polytechnic, Mencken's
    attendance at, 7
Bathing, of infant, 67, 72–73
Beer, effect on breastfeeding, 91–92
Behring, von, Emil, 141
Biedert, Philip, 95–96
Birth. *See also* Childbirth
    baby's shrill cry at, 47
Birthing suite, 53
"Black measles," 176
Bleeding, in treatment of
    pneumonia, 170
Blindness, ophthalmia neonatorum
    and, 50
Blood poisoning, in mother, 46,
    49–50

Boracic acid, as antiseptic, 74, 81
Bordet, Jules, 161
Bottlefeeding, 85–88. *See also* Formulas
   versus breastfeeding, 74–84, 92–97
Bottles, sterilization of, 99
Bouncing, of babies, 28
Brazelton, T. Berry, concept of infant capable of thought, 61
Breast(s), engorgement of, breastfeeding and, 70
Breastfeeding, 65–73, 74–84, 92–97
   advantages of, 69–70, 82–83
   contraindications to, 75, 77–78
   alcohol consumption and, 91, 97
   caffeine and, 92
   drugs and, 91
   immunologic benefits of, 79, 98
   jaundice and, 51
   medications incompatible with, 80
   mother's diet and, 75–76, 82–83
   mother's supply of milk for, effect of physical or mental disturbances on, 75, 79–80
   passive immunity and, 75
   schedule for, 66, 69
   trends in, 78–79
   versus bottlefeeding, 74–84, 92–97
   weaning from 106
   superstitions and fallacies about, 91–92
Breast milk, freezing of, 70
   freshness of, "fingernail technique" for analyzing, 93
   immunologic properties of, 75, 98
   pump for, 70
Breathing, brief cessation of (apnea), 43
   pattern of, in newborn infant, 46
Bright's disease (chronic kidney failure), in scarlet fever, 151
Broadway Magazine, Dreiser's success with, 4
Bubonic plague, 129
"Buck teeth," thumbsucking and, 42
Butterick, Ebenezer, 2
Butterick Company, distribution of baby book by, 15
   publications of, 2–3

Butterick Company *(continued)*
   sponsorship of schools for mothers, 6

CAFFEINE, breastfeeding and, 92, 97–98
   hyperactivity in infant and, 98
Casein, in cow's milk versus mother's milk, 85–86
Chapin, Charles, 108
Checkups, for babies, frequency of, 38–39
Chesney, Alan Mason, 22
Chickenpox, contagiousness of, 152
Childbed fever, in mother, 46, 49–50
Childbirth, dangers of, 46
   at home versus in hospital, 53
   role of midwives in, 53–54
Child care, information about, for parents, 51–52
Child Rescue Campaign, *Delineator's*, 5, 59
Childhood, communicable diseases of, 125–132
Children, White House Conference on, first, 5
   growing, food for, 105–110
Children's Bureau, address of, 52
   establishment of, 5
Chlamydia conjunctivitis, mother-to-infant transmission of, 50
Cholera, quarantines for, 129–130
Cigarette smoking, during pregnancy, 80
Clothing, for infants, 34
   selection of, 63
Coddling, of babies, 33, 34
Coffee, effect on breastfeeding, 92
Colic, 31–32
   type of cry associated with, 56
"Consumption," 75, 81. *See also* Tuberculosis
Colostrum, 69
Communicable diseases, 125–132
Cough, whooping, 156–164. *See also* Pertussis
Cow's milk. *See also* Bottlefeeding
   bacteria in, 86–87
   cost of, 103
   modification of, 32
Crisis of pneumonia, 166, 167, 171

Cry, colic-associated, 56
  shrill, at birth, 47
Crying, duration of, in healthy babies, 47
  nighttime, 32
  patterns of, in infants, 56–60

DEATH. *See* Mortality
Dehydration, urine color and, 69
The Delineator Magazine, 2–3, 4, 5, 13, 15
  Child Rescue Campaign of, 5, 59
  "If I Were Santa Claus" feature of, 6
Delivery, of infant. *See also* Birth; Childbirth
  midwives and, 53–54
Delivery room, father in, 53
The Designer, 2
Developmental milestones, achievement of, 57–59, 60–61
Diarrhea, 40, 41
  causes of, 99–100
Dick, George and Gladys, 153
Diet, as determinant of personality ("you are what you eat"), 89
  of nursing mother, 82–83
  for one-year-old infant, 88
Diphtheria, 133–144
  antitoxin for, 133–137, 141, 142, 143
  isolation of patient with, 138–139
  prevention of, 139
  vaccine for, development of, 142
Diphtheria/pertussis/tetanus (DPT) vaccine, 40
Disease(s), communicable, 125–132
  deadly, of infants, 1910 versus now, 40
  germ theory of, 127–128
  humoralism concept of, 126–127
  solidism theory of, 127
Doctor visits, for infants, frequency of, 38–39
Doubleday, Frank, *Sister Carrie* and, 3
Doubleday and Page, in battle over *Sister Carrie*, 3
Dreiser, Theodore, campaigns for child welfare, 4
  early career of, 3
  as editor of *Delineator*, 4

Dreiser, Theodore *(continued)*
  Hirshberg and, 18–19
  journalism career of, 3–4
  Mencken and, 1, 23
    first meeting of, 13–14
  "nervous breakdown" of, 3
  President Theodore Roosevelt and, 5
  Sister Carrie and, 3
DPT (diphtheria, pertussis, tetanus) vaccine, 40
Drugs, chemicals and, effect on breastfeeding, 80, 91
Durgin, Samuel, 116

EDUCATION, formal, Mencken's bias against, 111–115, 118
  Jesuit style of, 119
Ehrlich, Paul, 141
Enoch Pratt Free Library, Mencken Collection at, xi, 10
Erythromycin, in prevention of eye infections, 50
Eye color, of infants, 57
Eye infections, in newborn infant, 46, 50
Eyes, watery, in measles, 177, 179

FATHER, in delivery room, 53
  role in child care, 44
Fetal alcohol syndrome, 97
Fever, childbed, in mother, 46, 49–50
  scarlet, 145–155
  sweating and, 176
"Fingernail technique," for analysis of freshness of breast milk, 93
Fishbein, Morris, 22
Fluid needs of infant, determination of, 69
Fontanels, in newborn infant, importance of, 50
Food. *See also* Diet; Nutrition
  for growing children, 105–110
  solid, introduction of, timing of, 109–110
Formula(s), infant, change of, 102
  refrigeration of, 103
  sterilization of, 42
  types of, 97, 101
  versus breastfeeding, 74–84

Frankel, Albert, 171
Fresh air, infant's need for, 35, 42
Fruit, in child's diet, 107

GADDESDEN, John of, 180
Gengou, Octave, 161
Germ theory of disease, 41, 127–128
"Germs." *See also* Bacteria; Bacterial infections
　as cause of infectious diseases, 41, 42
　in cow's milk, 86–87
German method (percentage method) of infant feeding, 96
Glomerulonephritis, poststreptococcal, 151
Goldberger, Joseph, 181
Grandmother's advice, versus physician's, 27–30

HAARDT, Sara Powell, 7
Hair color, of infants, 57
Handwashing, importance of, in preventing spread of infection, 49–50
　poor, in spread of infectious diseases, 42
Head, shape of, in newborn infant, 46
Heart rate, of infant, 58
"Herd immunity," against measles, 182
Hippocrates, 170
Hirshberg, Leonard K., attendance at Johns Hopkins Medical School, 9
　"blind pool" scandal and, 20
　denouncement of, by Johns Hopkins Medical School, 23
　described by Fulton Oursler, 10, 17–18
　Dreiser and, 18–19
　fate of, 18–23
　first meeting with Mencken, 9
　Fulton Oursler's relationship to, 20–21
Hoffman, Arthur Sullivant, 2
Holt, L. Emmett, 43, 68, 77, 78, 82, 96, 109, 116
　The Care and Feeding of Children by, 16

Holt, L. Emmett *(continued)*
　A Catechism for Nurses by, 16
　Diseases of Infancy and Childhood by, 17
　works by, as models for Mencken's baby book, 13–17
Home remedies, avoidance of, 29–36
Humoralism, in concept of disease, 126–127
Hyperactivity, in infant, relationship to caffeine consumption by nursing mother, 98
Hyperbilirubinemia. *See* Jaundice

IMMUNITY, "herd," against measles, 182
　passive, breastfeeding and, 69–70
Infant, bathing of, 67, 72–73
　breastfeeding versus bottlefeeding of, 65–73, 74–84, 92–97
　breathing pattern of, 46
　clothing for, 34, 63
　"cost" of, 37
　crying patterns in, 59–60
　feeding of, current recommendations for, 109–110
　first few months of, 56–64
　first smile of, age at, 58
　intelligence of, development of, 58, 71
　newborn. *See* Baby; Newborn infant
　one-year-old, diet for, 88
　perception of pain by, 61
　playing with, 65, 68
　rigid schedule for, 63, 71
　sleeping pattern of, 68
　thinking, concept of, 61
　unthinking concept of, 56, 61, 65, 68
Infant mortality, 1910 versus 1980s, 39–41
Infant nutrition. *See also* Breastfeeding
　brief history of, 92–97
Infections, bacterial, management of, 41
　effect of breastfeeding on, 79

Infectious diseases, 125–132. *See also* specific types, e.g., Diphtheria
   prevention and treatment of, in 1910, 131–132
   spread of, poor handwashing and, 42
   susceptibility to, 152
   virulence in, 152
Intelligence, in infant, dawning of, 58
   development of, 71
Ipecac, 28
Itching, measles and, 176

JAUNDICE, breastfeeding and, 50–51
   in newborn infant, 46–47, 50–51
Jennie Gerhardt, Mencken's review of, 3
Jesuit style of education, 119
Johns Hopkins Medical School, Hirshberg and, 9, 22–23
Journal of the American Medical Association, exposé of Hirshberg, 23

KIDNEY failure, chronic, scarlet fever and, 151
Kissing, of baby, warning against, 33, 65, 68, 70–71
   in spread of diphtheria, 139
Knopf, Alfred A., 22
Koch's postulates of disease, 128, 152, 153, 161
Koplik's spots, in measles, 175, 181

LAENNEC, R.T.H., 170

MEASLES, 174–184
   "black," 176
   "herd immunity" against, 182
   itching and, 176
   vaccine for, 40, 181–182
   watery eyes and, 177, 179
Meat, in child's diet, 106–107
Meat Inspection Act of 1907, 95
Medical advice, expert, 29, 36, 37
Medications, effect on expectant or breastfeeding mothers, 80
Mencken, August, 7
Mencken, Henry Louis, attendance at Baltimore Polytechnic, 7

Mencken, Henry Louis *(continued)*
   employment at his father's cigar factory, 7
   hatred for quackery, 22
   Hirshberg and, 9, 19, 21–22
   last years of, 23–24
   marriage to Sara Powell Haardt, 7
   Newspaper Days and, 8
   review of *Jennie Gerhardt*, 3
   school days of, 7, 117–118
   Theodore Dreiser and, 1, 23
      first meeting of, 13–14
Mencken Collection, at Enoch Pratt Free Library in Baltimore, xi, 10
Meningitis, 41
Midwives, role in childbirth, 53–54
Milestones, developmental, achievement of, 57–59, 60–61
Milk, bacteria in, 41–42
   breast. *See* Breast milk
   chapter on, 89–92
   in child's diet, 106–108
   cow's. *See* Cow's milk
   handling of, in early 1900s, 41–42
   mother's. *See* Breastfeeding
   pasteurization of, definition of, 102
   refrigeration of, 103
   "tainted," prior to refrigeration, 95
MMR (measles, mumps, rubella) vaccine, 40
Morgagni, Giovanni, 127
Morse, Moreau, 116
Mortality, infant, 1910 versus 1980s, 39–41
Mother(s), childbed fever in, 46, 449–450
   nursing, diet of, 75–76, 82–83
   superstitions of, in care of infants, 29, 40
   of young babies, common mistake of, 83
Mouth, grayish-white spots on mucosa of, as precursor to measles, 175, 181
Mouth breathing, 42, 43
Mumps, vaccine for, 40

NAPS, daytime, 71
Newborn infant, 45–55. *See also* Baby; Infant

Newborn infant *(continued)*
   average weight of, 46
   breathing pattern in, 46
   eye infections in, 46, 50
   head shape of, 46
   intelligence of, 47
   jaundice in, 46–47, 50–51
   movements of, 57
   need for sleep, 65, 71
   shedding of skin by, 47
   shedding of tears by, 47, 51
   skull development of, 50
   typical appearance of, 46–47
   weight loss by, in first days of life, 78
New Idea Women's Magazine, 2
Newspaper Days, Mencken and, 8
Nurse, good, theme of, in Mencken's works, 153
Nurse-midwife, role in childbirth, 53–54
Nursing. *See* Breastfeeding
Nursing mother, alcohol consumption and, 97
   diet of, 75–76, 82–83
   superstitions about, 91–92
Nutrition, good, in prevention of disease, 42
   infant. *See also* Breastfeeding
   brief history of, 92–97

Oliver Optic, 112
Ophthalmia neonatorum, blindness and, 50
Oral mucosa, grayish-white spots on, as precursor to measles; 175, 181
Orphans, *Delineator's* Child Rescue Campaign for, 5
Osler, Sir William, 36, 169
Oursler, Fulton, description of Hirshberg, 10, 18–19
   relationship to Hirshberg, 20–21

Pacifiers, 28, 29, 42
Pain, infant's perception of, 61–62
Palladino, Eusapia, role in Dreiser-Hirshberg rift, 18–19
Panum, Peter Ludwig, 180
Pap, panada and, as baby food, 94
Paregoric, 33

Parenting classes, obtaining information about, 52
Parenting skills, acquisition of, 45, 48, 51–52
Passive immunity, breastfeeding and, 75
Pasteur, Louis, pasteurization of milk and, 90, 95
Pasteurization, definition of, 102
   of milk, 90, 95
Patent medicines, avoidance of, 29–36
Pediatrician(s), advice of, versus grandmother's, 29, 36
   educational requirements for, 48–49
   number of, in U.S., 49
   selection of, 44–46, 48–49, 53
   questions to ask in, 49
Percentage method of infant feeding, 96
Personality, development of, 105
Pertussis. *See also* Whooping cough
   vaccine for, 161
      adverse effects of, 161–162
      position of American Academy of Pediatrics on, 161–162
Physical examinations, for babies, frequency of, 38–39
Physician's advice, versus grandmother's, 29, 36
Playing, with infant, 65, 68
Pneumonia, 165–174
   community-acquired versus hospital acquired, 171
   as complication of measles, 179
   as complication of whooping cough, 158
   crisis in, 171
Poliomyelitis vaccine, 40
Poststreptococcal glomerulonephritis, 151
Pott's disease (tuberculosis of spine), 75, 81–82
Powers, Grover, 96
Pratt Library, in Baltimore, Mencken Collection of, xi, 10
Pregnancy, alcohol consumption during, 97
   cigarette smoking during, 80

Prenatal care, importance of, 40, 52
Prenatal conferences, in selecting a pediatrician, 49
Progressive Era, magazines of, 2
"Pseudo-diphtheria," 140, 141
Pure Food and Drug Act of 1906, 95

QUARANTINES, origin of, 128–129
   for cholera, 129–130
   for tuberculosis, 130

RAMON, Gaston, 142
Rash, in measles, 175
   in measles versus scarlet fever, 180
   in scarlet fever, 146, 150
"Raspberry" tongue, of scarlet fever, 146
Recess, introduction into school curriculum, 120
Refrigeration, absence of, effect on milk, 41–42
Rhazes, 179
Rheumatic fever, scarlet fever and, 150
Rocking the baby, 65, 68
Rokitansky, von, Carl, 170
Roosevelt, President Theodore, Dreiser's meeting with, 5
Rotch, Thomas Morgan, 96
Roux, Pierre, 141
Rubella vaccine, 40

SAGE of Baltimore. *See* Mencken, Henry Louis
St. Vitus's dance (chorea), 30, 35, 44
Scarlet fever, 145–155
   differentiated from measles, 151
   rheumatic fever as sequel to, 150
Schedule, rigid, for infants, 63, 71
School days, Mencken's, 117–118
School phobia, 119
School sickness, 111, 118–119
School(s), adverse effects of, Mencken's view of, 111–115
   assessment of, by parents, 121–122
   deficits of, how to deal with, 122
   ideal age for starting, Mencken's view of, 112, 115

School(s), *(continued)*
   importance of recess from, 119–120
   medical inspections of, 116–117
   poor conditions in, in early 1900s, 114
   and school-related problems, 111–124
Semmelweis, Ignaz P., 49–50
Simon, Franz, 95–96
Sister Carrie, 3
Skin, shedding of, by newborn infant, 47
Skull, development of, 50
Sleep, infant's need for, 65, 71
   infant's pattern of, 32, 36, 68
Sleep apnea, 43
Small pox, 179, 180
Smile, first, age at, 58
Smith's Magazine, Dreiser as editor of, 4
Smoking, during pregnancy, 80
Solid foods, introduction of, timing of, 109–110
Solidism, in concept of disease, 127
Soxhlet's sterilization process, for milk, 90, 95
Spinal tuberculosis, 75, 81, 82
Spock, Benjamin, 16, 17
Spots, Koplik's, in measles, 175
Sterilization, of bottles and nipples, importance of, 99
   of infant formulas and drinking water, 42
Stethoscope, invention of, 170
"Strep throat," 41
Streptococcus pyogenes, as cause of scarlet fever, 153
Superstitions, mothers', in care of infants, 29, 40
   about nursing mothers, 91–92
Sweating, fever and, 176
Sydenham, Thomas, 151, 180

TABULA *rasa* (blank slate), concept of, 56, 61, 65, 68
Talking, age of onset of, 58
Tea, effect on breastfeeding, 92
Tears, shedding of, by newborn infant, 47, 51

Teething, 28, 37
  age at onset of, 58
Thumbsucking, 42
Toddlers, feeding of, current recommendations for, 109–110
Tongue, raspberry appearance of, in scarlet fever, 146
Tonsils, removal of, 43
Tuberculosis, children with, school attendance and, 122–123
  as contraindication to breastfeeding, 75, 81
  of spine, 75, 81–82

URINE color, as indicator of dehydration, 69

VACCINATIONS, 40–41
Vaccine, diphtheria, development of, 142
  measles, 181–182
  pertussis, 161
Vegetables, in child's diet, 107
Virulence, in infectious diseases, 152
Virchow, Rudolph, 127
Vomiting, causes of, 100

WALKERS, for infants, 59, 62
Walking, age of onset of, 58–59
Walking aids, for infants, 59, 62
Water, baby's need for, 67, 69
Weaning, from breastfeeding, 106
Weight, average, of newborn baby, 46
  loss of, in first days of life, 78
Well-child care, 38–39
Wet nurses, 82, 94
What You Ought To Know About Your Baby, origin of book, 12–18
White House Conference on Children, first, 5
Whooping cough, 156–164
Wilder, George, 2
  hiring of Dreiser, 4
  influence of Holt's pediatric book on, 16–17
  interest in infant crying patterns, 59
  role in baby book, 6, 14, 15

YELLOW color, in newborn infant, 46–47, 51

Please send me _____ copies of

Markel/Oski:

The H. L. Mencken Baby Book

Price: $18.95 (includes postage & handling)

I enclose payment: ☐ Check   ☐ Visa   ☐ MasterCard

Credit Card # _____

Expiration Date _____

Signature _____

Name _____

Address _____

City/State/Zip _____

Please send me _____ copies of

Markel/Oski:

The H. L. Mencken Baby Book

Price: $18.95 (includes postage & handling)

I enclose payment: ☐ Check   ☐ Visa   ☐ MasterCard

Credit Card # _____

Expiration Date _____

Signature _____

Name _____

Address _____

City/State/Zip _____

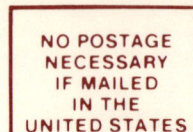

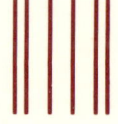

BUSINESS REPLY CARD
FIRST CLASS   PERMIT NO. 33107   PHILADELPHIA, PA

POSTAGE WILL BE PAID BY ADDRESSEE

NO POSTAGE
NECESSARY
IF MAILED
IN THE
UNITED STATES

HANLEY & BELFUS, INC.
Medical Publishers
P.O. Box 1377
Philadelphia, PA 19105-9990

BUSINESS REPLY CARD
FIRST CLASS   PERMIT NO. 33107   PHILADELPHIA, PA

POSTAGE WILL BE PAID BY ADDRESSEE

NO POSTAGE
NECESSARY
IF MAILED
IN THE
UNITED STATES

HANLEY & BELFUS, INC.
Medical Publishers
P.O. Box 1377
Philadelphia, PA 19105-9990